The Disease of Belief

How Your Convictions Can Heal You or Destroy You

Kevin Hoffarth, MD, IFMCP

ISBN: 978-1-970757-00-2

ACKNOWLEDGEMENTS

To my wife — the strongest person I know. You carry grace when I am at my weakest and show me, every single day, what unconditional love truly looks like.

To my daughter, Charlie — who chose to be my daughter and, in doing so, gave me the greatest gift of all: the privilege of experiencing fatherhood in its truest, most beautiful form.

To every soul who has allowed me the honor of walking beside them as their physician and guide — thank you. I have learned far more from you than you could ever imagine, and your courage continues to inspire my own.

To my Starbucks A-team — thank you for greeting me each morning with a smile, a perfectly brewed cup of coffee, and just the right dose of banter. You've turned a simple daily ritual into a sanctuary of connection and joy.

And to all my friends and colleagues who continue to raise the collective consciousness in health and medicine — you know who you are. It is an honor to walk this shared path of awakening, discovery, and evolution with each of you.

Table of Contents

CHAPTER 1

From Glowing Stoves to Quantum Leaps

By the end of the 1800s, physicists believed they were close to fully understanding the universe. Building on the work of **Newton** and **Maxwell**, they had created a framework known as **classical physics**, which explained everything from planetary motion to the behavior of light. To them, the world seemed **predictable** and nearly complete, with all the great discoveries already made.

Yet a closer look at something as ordinary as stovetop coils heating and glowing exposed a serious flaw. Classical physics predicted that the hotter an object became, the brighter it would glow and the more energy it would release as light. The math worked perfectly for low-energy light, like infrared or red. However, when the same equations were extended to higher-energy light, such as ultraviolet and beyond, the math collapsed, spiraling into infinity.

This was a crisis for physics.

According to those equations, heating any metal object with increasingly higher energy, like the stovetop coil, would cause it to radiate limitless energy, eventually releasing an infinite amount of radiation. Of course, if that were true, everything in your kitchen would instantly vaporize.

This mismatch between theory and reality became known as the **"Ultraviolet Catastrophe."** What physicists once believed to be a complete understanding of the universe turned out to have fundamental flaws.

The Quantum Leap

Enter Max Planck.

In 1900, Planck took a radical step. Rather than viewing energy as smooth and continuous, he proposed it came in indivisible packets called **quanta**. That one leap aligned the math with reality, explaining the glowing stove and giving birth to **quantum physics**.

Planck opened the door, and Einstein, Bohr, Schrödinger, Heisenberg, and many others rushed in. They revealed a universe that is **much stranger** and more alive than anyone had imagined: light acting as both a wave and a particle, electrons jumping in **quantized orbits**, and reality shimmering as **probabilities** until it is observed. The rigid, clockwork universe gave way to a dynamic **field of possibilities**. It also required a completely new math (a new language) based on linear algebra and complex equations.

The 'Catastrophe' of Medicine Today

But here's the profound truth: this fundamental misunderstanding isn't isolated to the study of physics. Medicine's progress and success have been limited by viewing health and disease solely through the lens of the <u>physical</u>. This narrow view has led to its own quiet catastrophe, the inability to heal most chronic diseases and model out a more decisive etiology to disease.

Ask most physicians today, **"Doctor, why me? Why did I get this disease?"** and the responses will vary from a slew of biochemical or anatomical explanations, all the way to "you were at higher risk," or the most authentic, "I don't know." The way in which Planck ushered in quantum thinking necessitates an appeal to medicine to apply its applications to healing, since quantum physics uncovers the essence of what we are made of.

For years, I practiced as I was trained, guided by protocols and checklists - the Maytag repairman of the human body. It worked until it didn't. Patients weren't fully healing, their symptoms returning. Health improvements remained stagnant. I started to see the limits of treating the body as a machine with broken parts. That realization led me to **Functional Medicine**, a discipline focused on root causes and interconnected systems. Making that leap felt like a paradigm shift akin to Planck's creation of the quanta. I was able to see the same information, now through a different lens which allowed me to view the body differently than how I was initially taught. Suddenly, disease and healing began to realign, though unfortunately, still with the same inherent flaws.

So, my journey didn't stop there.

As I explored genetics, epigenetics, energy, neuro-immune-endocrinology, meditation, and quantum physics, among other fields, I realized even more clearly that true healing doesn't come solely from the body or environment; it exists in the mind, within our thoughts. That realization led me to **Biological Decoding**, which understands that symptoms are not just biological but also a language that expresses unresolved emotions and hidden conflicts written into the body, linking emotional issues to specific organ problems.

This is the heart of my book.

We have been taught to believe that health problems are solely the result of our physical bodies breaking down. For example, we assume that heart disease happens because of poor physical choices like eating unhealthy food, not exercising, or having "bad genes." We see the world in simple cause-and-effect terms, much like the early classical physicists did, until their math eventually failed when pushed too far.

Medicine, when confined to traditional boundaries, also breaks down. Why does one person who follows all the rules—eating well, exercising, keeping their cholesterol in check—still suffer a heart attack at age 45, while another who eats poorly, never exercises, and smokes lives to 95? When our patients ask the critical question, **"Why me? Why did I get this disease?"**, conventional medicine often can't provide a satisfying answer. However, when we apply quantum-level thinking to medicine, using the model of Biological Decoding that has existed since at least the 1980s, the math begins to align again, just as it did when quanta were first described.

Applying the scientific understanding of our non-physical world from our quantum physicist colleagues helps us better address the complex questions in medicine that we all ask. However, as a physician, I can tell you it's incredibly uncomfortable because it also eliminates the simplicity of cause and effect as our explanation for patients, replacing it with a realm of predictability based on probability. Neither patient nor physician enjoys viewing disease through this lens. Yet, I will demonstrate in this book that it is precisely what we all need to start doing, and the great news is that it empowers each person to realize that the starting point, and even the potential solution, of disease begins and ends with us.

Many of our beliefs are inherited stories that shape our choices and decisions, but they can also disrupt the mind's harmony with the body's natural rhythm and, if left unchecked, lead to disease. Once we recognize the patterns that hold us back, we see that those beliefs and thoughts which have been linked to strong emotions become subconscious background programs that quietly influence our biology without us realizing it. When we mistake these beliefs for fixed facts, they limit and weaken us, often at the expense of our health. However, when we bring them into awareness, they can be rewritten, allowing our biology to return to its natural, optimal flow.

This book is about **gathering the many puzzle pieces of our health**—social media posts, news articles, podcasts, your doctor's advice, medical journals, and the stories of loved ones, and organizing them into a picture poised for the kinds of questions that challenge today's current boundaries of medicine more fully. It will also help better address the questions we all ask when illness strikes: *"Why me? What caused my disease?"*

The way I teach and share throughout this book emphasizes one truth: you are not fixed by genetics, bound by destiny, or doomed to repeat past stories. Like Planck staring at a glowing stove, we must question the inherited "equations" of medicine and let go of the ones that no longer fit.

What seems ordinary: a thought, a belief, or a moment of awareness, can either open new realities or close the door completely; only you decide its fate. **My goal is to expand your mind with the intent to make you uncomfortable and leave you with an unquenchable desire to keep learning.** Once you accept that, a whole new version of your own understanding about life will emerge.

Each of us unconsciously carries **"diseases of belief"** that fracture our relationships, limit our experiences, and can even shape our biology toward illness. This book will invite you to explore your emotional outlook, question your beliefs, and expand your perspective. Along the way, I'll offer thought-provoking **"Rabbit Holes,"** seeds of curiosity designed to challenge your patterns of belief and make you feel uncomfortable, intentionally. These seeds fall outside the realm of this book. While they don't necessarily represent my beliefs, they do test your ability to sit with discomfort and see beyond your own belief paradigms.

The more flexible your thinking, the freer your biology becomes. **If an idea hits a nerve, lean into it.** Your ego will try to protect you by pulling away, but resistance only hinders growth in thought. This book challenges you to cultivate curiosity, engage in self-reflection, and develop humility. Get used to saying, *"I don't know, but I'm willing to ask questions, listen openly, and potentially move beyond my current belief limits."*

Writing this book was difficult for the same reasons that quantum mechanics was challenging for early physicists—its subject matter is abstract. The laws of the quantum world are based on probabilities rather than certainties, which makes them deeply unsettling, just like thoughts and emotions create deep uncertainty for healthcare providers.

We are emotional beings shaped by the long story of who we are and that story also influences our biology. The goal here is to help you reconnect with your story, examine the emotions that affect your health and inner peace, and identify where they *might* be fueling disease today. As you go through this journey of self-discovery, you'll gain a new and deeper perspective on life. I want you to take pride in being your own CEO, **living from your most authentic self, one that reflects your true beliefs rather than those inherited.**

This non-physical dimension of health begins and ends with your beliefs.

If you're ready to examine your emotional landscape, let this book guide you. Together, we will uncover the hidden costs of unresolved emotions and rewrite the story of your health, one thought at a time.

CHAPTER 2

BREAKING THE CHAINS OF CONVENTIONAL MEDICINE

I wear many hats, but at the heart of them all is my role as a physician guide, planting small "seeds" of thought that grow over time. My passion is helping patients not just survive but truly thrive. Over the years, I've been privileged to walk alongside thousands of people as they navigate the unpredictable journey we call Life.

In 2011, I was introduced to Functional Medicine by one of my Earth Angels, Amy Beth Hopkins, a physical therapist and someone who planted an enormous seed in *my* life that grew into a robust oak. She read one of my notes for a shared patient and said, "You know, when I read your notes, you sound like a Functional Medicine physician." At the time, I wasn't sure if that was a compliment. I asked her what she meant, and like any good teacher, she encouraged me to experience it for myself. That day, I signed up for the next Functional Medicine conference, which happened to be in Denver, CO.

After my first day of lectures, two things became clear. First, I found a community of physicians also searching for missing links to improve patient care. Second, I was completely overwhelmed. I remember calling my wife after my first eight hours of lectures, forgetting I was sharing an elevator with six other attendees. I said loudly, "I have no idea what these people are talking about. I feel like the dumbest person in the room. They are speaking another language. It's like I never went to medical school." I was so absorbed in my own reptilian brain panic that I didn't realize everyone in the elevator heard me, and a big laugh erupted. Each person shared that they had felt the same way when first learning to think like a Functional Medicine provider. That reassurance became a turning point, and I never felt that kind of overwhelm in the same way again with Functional Medicine.

Until that day, my training had been rooted in traditional Western allopathic medicine, focused primarily on diagnosing and treating symptoms with pharmaceuticals. But on that day, I was introduced to a new way of thinking, and I couldn't unsee it. I felt as though I stood at a massive crossroads, a moment I will later describe as my second midlife crisis. My heart could no longer justify simply managing disease. I aimed to promote healing, so I chose to embrace Functional Medicine. I knew in my heart that this discovery would fundamentally alter who I was as a physician.

Let me be crystal clear...

Functional Medicine is not a new medicine; it is a framework of thought that better encompasses all the factors contributing to the origin of *physical* disease. It empowers us to reverse engineer disease in ways traditional medicine does not.

In my first book, **Functional Medicine: The New Standard**, I described how medical school trained me to view disease through a narrow lens, focusing only on the final chapters of the "Book of Disease." Functional medicine helped me resolve those earlier chapters that led to disease. I shared ways humans can support their physical health using the acronym **S.T.A.M.P** (Stressors, Toxins, Allergens, Microbes, and Poor Diet). By addressing these triggers that compromise our physical barrier linings (i.e., the mucosa of our gut, lungs, brain, and skin), we minimize activation and, more importantly, the prolonged over-activation of our immune system, the root *physical* driver of disease. This book received a warm welcome from readers, many of whom have gotten sick, so to speak, of America's existing consumer healthcare system. I advocated for a proactive approach, promoting what the miraculous human body is inherently designed to do.

Since publishing my first book, I have spent a lot of time exploring the idea that there are earlier chapters in the "Book of Disease" that occur prior to the **S.T.A.M.P. triggers.** This idea challenged the notion that only the physical heals the physical. However, as I researched further, I realized this required a new way of thinking

19

and a revised language to help make the connection between the physical and the non-physical for patient and physician understanding as well as application.

Functional Medicine offers a mental framework for understanding the *physical* causes of disease and how to effectively address them. However, I always tell my new patients that my other goal is to help them **"get out of their own way."** This involves navigating a more abstract, non-physical realm that includes their disease of beliefs—their thoughts that have been linked to deeply rooted emotions. For this, I needed a framework as logical and structured as Functional Medicine but flexible enough to work within the realm of quantum thinking, where we deal with the immaterial, the world of possibility and probabilities.

Let me be crystal clear again...

Functional Medicine does not have all the answers. What it offers is a valuable mental framework that clarifies connections between different medical domains. Yet, if we confine ourselves to this single framework, we risk creating just another "Disease of Belief," limiting our ability to think expansively in the world of the non-physical. Discomfort in thought is a catalyst for growth, and this book will challenge your comfort zone as much as it has challenged mine.

This is where Biological Decoding comes in.

Biological Decoding parallels the journey of Functional Medicine from 30 years ago. It is reshaping our understanding of disease, yet is still not widely accepted or appreciated. It explores the emotional and psychological roots of illness by tracing conditions back to original thoughts, emotions, or unresolved subconscious conflicts.

Its theoretical foundation goes back centuries, as humans have sought to see illness as more than just the result of external or inherited factors. Pioneers such as William James, Claude Bernard, and Carl Lange investigated the relationship between emotions and internal balance, laying the groundwork for the **field of psychosomatic medicine**. Walter Cannon and Hans Selye expanded our knowledge of stress and its physiological effects, while Konrad Lorenz and Henri Laborit investigated instinctive and learned responses to trauma. These ideas came together in fields such as psychoneuroimmunology, neuroscience, and transgenerational studies, **connecting emotional experiences to physical symptoms.**

In the early 1980s, like Planck, Dr. Ryke Geerd Hamer made a daring quantum leap in thought, born out of unbearable loss. In August 1978, his nineteen-year-old son was accidentally shot by a friend. Four months later, his son died. The grief was crushing, a wound no parent should ever have to endure. And then, as if tragedy had not already taken enough, Hamer himself was diagnosed with testicular cancer just months later, at the age of forty-three.

The timing haunted him. Could his own cancer be connected to the trauma of losing his son? Was this more than mere coincidence? That question consumed him. He began interviewing cancer patients, searching for patterns, and what he found was uncanny. Time and again, patients shared stories of shocks, losses, betrayals, and moments of deep emotional trauma that seemed to precede their illness. Hamer wondered if the body, like the mind, stored these wounds, transforming emotional conflicts into physical disease.

At the University of Munich, he went further, interviewing thousands of patients. A striking theme emerged: **specific conflicts seemed to strike specific organs**. The testicles, in biological terms, are symbols of creation, fertility, and lineage, linking a man's identity to his child. In testicular cancer patients, the recurring story was profound loss: a child gone, a partner lost, or a future legacy suddenly threatened. From the lens of Biological Decoding, testicular cancer could be seen as the body's unconscious attempt to "replace" or "make up for" what had been lost.

And here lies one of the central principles of this book: the mind does not clearly distinguish between thought and reality. To the mind, the signal was simple, more testicular cells are needed. The body responded by producing them rapidly, and the world gave that process a name: cancer.

From these insights, Hamer built what he would call New German Medicine, a radical idea that every disease begins with a deep, isolating shock, a moment so intense it sends shockwaves through the psyche, the brain, and into a specific organ.

It was a bold vision...and bold visions rarely find easy acceptance. Hamer was shunned, his medical license stripped away. He was branded a heretic. Yet history is full of such stories. John Snow (1813-1858), once dismissed as eccentric for removing the Broad Street pump handle, ultimately proved that cholera spread through contaminated water and became the father of modern epidemiology. Joseph Lister (1827-1912), mocked for spraying carbolic acid in the operating room, revolutionized surgery with antiseptic technique, saving countless lives.

Hamer's story, too, begins in rejection. But as history has shown us, ideas born in exile sometimes carry the seeds of transformation.

Science is not just a body of knowledge but a series of continuing questions. Dr. Hamer's quantum leap connecting emotional conflict to a specific organ inspired many others to expand on his groundbreaking work. Today, many are unknowingly refining it, with each contribution adding to the puzzle that has led to today's new thought paradigm: Biological

Decoding.

Dr. Bernard Sabbah expanded the understanding of the subconscious, demonstrating how deeply-rooted emotions influence disease processes. Later work by Marc Fréchet, Boris Cyrulnik, and Carl Jung built on this foundation.

Today, Isabelle Benarous has integrated these ideas with therapeutic approaches, including neurolinguistic programming (NLP) and BioReprogramming, to turn Biological Decoding from a theoretical concept into practical healing methods. Isabelle is my latest Earth Angel, who planted the seed of Biological Decoding in my life. That seed continues to grow, just like Amy Beth's seed of Functional Medicine, guiding me in applying these tools and principles practically and meaningfully.

The historical foundation of Biological Decoding has been reinforced, albeit unknowingly, by modern thought leaders such as Dr. Joe Dispenza, Dr. Bruce Lipton, Dr. Tara Swart, Deepak Chopra, Wayne Dyer, and Gregg Braden. Together, their work highlights the influence of thoughts and beliefs on physical biology, creating a link between scientific principles and mind-body medicine.

As I explained in *Functional Medicine: The New Standard*, disease is like a book written across many chapters. Western medicine usually enters near the final chapters, treating advanced disease with the aim of managing symptoms and slowing progression. Functional Medicine turns the pages back, looking to the earlier chapters to identify the **S.T.A.M.P triggers** that set dysfunction in motion. Biological Decoding reaches even further, into the opening chapters, searching for the potential smoking gun behind why disease arises in the first place. It examines the potential initiating triggers, often unresolved emotional conflicts, shaped by what I call: **The Disease of Belief**, which silently influences our physical outcomes. Within this framework, health and illness are seen as creative acts born from thought, often unconscious, existing in the quantum space where energy, emotion, and biology converge. It is a realm that can feel both fascinating and murky, and, at times, deeply uncomfortable.

When we hold strong beliefs, which are simply thoughts connected to deeply rooted emotions, they are often buried symbolically in our subconscious. I will explain how they exert a powerful influence on our physical health. This book adds many puzzle pieces, developed in the 21st century, to show how our thoughts and emotions impact our physical biology, offering the clearest insight into the origin of disease I have come across to better guide those who ask, **"Why me? What caused my disease?"**

This leads to understanding health and disease beyond the physical. If we don't release our conflicts and instead suppress them, we keep carrying them in our psyche, like adding bricks to a backpack. I will show you how these metaphorical bricks represent the diseases of belief—conflicts of thoughts and emotions stored in our bodies causing us to develop disease in response to our unresolved issues within specific organs, as Dr. Hamer first attempted to demonstrate.

In my practice, patients who have surpassed their physical health goals still need to progress to the next stage of wellness. They have completed the "undergraduate course" of understanding the **S.T.A.M.P. triggers,** but must pursue the "Ph.D. program."

In this advanced degree program, they gradually realize that their beliefs, which are thoughts connected to deeply rooted emotions, can influence disease development if left unchecked. Without exploring this deeper level of health, even my top physical performers remain vulnerable to inner turmoil and, as a result, illness. I will include several examples in this book of patients who were physically 'doing everything right' but still developed physical illness. Biological Decoding offers a thought template for both patients and providers to better navigate the often-unclear world of thoughts and emotions.

Take me, for example.

At 53, I am in excellent physical shape. My DEXA scans place me in the top 1% for my age group, and my biomarkers are optimized. Yet, by age 40, my autoimmune disease, ankylosing spondylitis, had already ravaged my lower spine. I believed I was doing everything right based on Western training, but Functional Medicine taught me to analyze each chapter of disease and understand why my body took this path.

By identifying my hidden triggers within the S.T.A.M.P. framework, I deactivated three sets of autoantibodies over a year. Still, my disease had been ongoing for as long as I could remember, and these physical triggers did not fully explain why my body initially chose this path. I knew I needed a different framework to look beneath the surface and understand my disease of beliefs, my origin story to the questions: "Why me? Why did I get this disease?"

Biological Decoding provided that thought framework. It revealed the origin story of my disease better than an explanation through Western medicine or Functional Medicine.

During the first seven years of our lives, we develop a powerful subconscious program, learning how to walk, how to eat, and even how to interact with others in a dynamic way. In these first seven years, our brain waves are primarily in a hypnosis-like state. We are literally sponges, absorbing this new information, not unlike a computer with newly installed software. However, once we learn to walk, we don't need to relearn it; it becomes an automatic process that works continuously and unconsciously in the background.

What oversees this expansive subconscious programming is our ego, whose main goal is self-protection. The ego was formed from a combination of many beliefs. Unfortunately, our emotional reactions to others are mainly defensive responses shaped by those who raised us and the beliefs we adopted. Additionally, we absorb our caretakers' beliefs during those first seven years without even realizing it. As a result, many of our beliefs, simply thoughts linked to deep-rooted emotions, are not even truly ours but downloaded programs. That's why it's essential to engage in mental gardening and weed out which beliefs are genuinely our own and which ones we've simply absorbed subconsciously. Those that don't align with us today often serve as subconscious triggers, with our ego in the driver's seat.

You must admit that this is empowering once you understand that, right?

The stiffness created by my ankylosing spondylitis occurred before I was a truly conscious human, meaning in the first seven years of my life. I know because I have never been able to sit on the ground in a "crisscross applesauce" position without falling over. It embarrassed me as early as I can remember anything.

In the first seven years of my life, my father was dealing with his own set of conflicts (as every parent does) that I later learned about. At that time, he had three young children, had recently finished his residency as an Ear, Nose, and Throat doctor, was managing my mom's emotional breakdowns (which I will share more about later), and they moved from Ohio to California to start a new medical practice. My father, like many men in their early 30s, felt overwhelmed by a flood of emotions. I am the youngest and the only son, so I subconsciously absorbed his programming that included his own conflicts, acting as his emotional support and foundation, placing him on a pedestal throughout my early years.

As I grew older, being his emotional support led to my own conflict, centered on our relationship and the ongoing emotional struggle of feeling responsible for supporting his emotional needs. Still, I did not make that connection until I personally met with Isabelle Benarous, one of the premier Biological Decoders in the US today. I often prioritized his needs over my own and acted as a steady, unwavering source of emotional support. For decades, I admired my dad while keeping myself small around him for his sake.

It is common for a son to assume this role for his father. For me, I subconsciously absorbed my father's inner conflicts, which arose from his feeling of carrying the weight of his entire family on his shoulders. Biologically, the parts of the body that primarily support carrying such heavy burdens are the spine and pelvis. As you will learn, beliefs contain built-in energy. If the emotions connected to them are deeply held and intense, the belief can hold significant energy, making it more impactful on the biology. Ankylosing spondylitis is an autoimmune disease that affects (and over time can damage) the lower part of the spine and the hip pelvis, which form the foundation of our skeletal structure.

If you look at an X-ray of my lower spine, it almost resembles a hard piece of bamboo: sturdy, firm, and unmoving, but that is not how it is supposed to appear. The vertebrae are designed to connect in a way that allows simple movements, such as leaning over to pick something up. Suppose my emotional conflict around my role in the family required me to be the emotional foundation for my father, holding the entire family on my *own* shoulders. In that case, my body would adapt by becoming more rigid and inflexible. We often view disease as something negative, but what if our body creates an environment in response to the input it receives? Your mind does not distinguish between your thoughts and reality; it simply sends signals that support the input. In this way, our body's physical structure results from a continuous stream of signals collected at the gene level, ultimately shaping our physical biology.

However, it was not just the downloading of his conflicts into my subconscious programming that caused my disease. That was my origin story, but its progression had to do with my own Disease of Beliefs, meaning that my beliefs, as I grew older, came into constant conflict with my dad's beliefs that I subconsciously absorbed early in my life. My father was my most powerful influencer, and therefore, in my early years, I downloaded his views on his generation's attitudes as well as his own beliefs toward paternalism, misogyny, and expressing love through guilt and shame.

It's common that, as people become thoughtful adults, the beliefs they unconsciously absorbed as children turn into emotional triggers, which are the result of our subconscious protector: our Ego. When my adult beliefs conflicted with the beliefs I inherited from my father, it led to the development of my own "Disease of Beliefs." These conflicts between my conscious mind, shaped by my life experiences, and the subconscious downloads of my father's beliefs continued to fuel the fire as I grew older, often unknowingly. Over the years, these conflicts brought more issues for me because they didn't align with my own downloaded beliefs, creating lots of emotional triggers around my father. These contradictions not only explain why I developed ankylosing spondylitis but also sustain the original flames. When these emotional conflicts interact with a body dealing with underlying **S.T.A.M.P. triggers**, each one intensifies the fire further, potentially causing the disease to progress.

Let me be crystal clear again.

How each of us interprets our thoughts and feelings is shaped by the lens of our personal story. This isn't about deciding what is right or wrong, true or false, but simply about what *is*. Perhaps the most important part of honoring your inner conflicts is learning not to judge them, but instead to observe them with curiosity. I call this the nebulous non-physical world because no two people perceive the same set of experiences in the same way. Once you truly accept this, for yourself and for others, you open both your mind and your heart.

I invite you to hold onto this framework as you read this book, even if you take away nothing else. It echoes one of the most curious lessons drawn from quantum physics: reality does not solidify until our attention collapses the possibilities into form. Put another way, as I mentioned in my last book: **"Where thoughts go, energy flows."**

As you read this book, a crucial first step is to become deeply aware of your own powerful emotional reactions, recognizing that they are closely tied to your beliefs. Adopt a curious, observer mindset by asking yourself, "What thought triggered this emotion?" Within the framework of Biological Decoding, which embraces the nonphysical, immaterial world of quantum thinking, grounded in probabilities rather than certainty, we come to understand that thoughts and emotions are not inherently 'good' or 'bad', instead, they reveal which thoughts create unresolved conflicts within your own consciousness and within the greater consciousness of all that exists.

Each person's perception of their experiences varies, and observing these conflicts with curiosity, without judgment, is the first step toward releasing them. Suppressed conflicts accumulate like bricks in a backpack, eventually manifesting as physical disease. My spine, rigid and immovable like bamboo, reflects my body's response to decades of unresolved emotional burdens that I initially downloaded during the creation of my own super subconscious.

When I look back at all the patients I have worked with over 25 years, I cannot think of a single **S.T.A.M.P. trigger** that explains a patient's disease thoroughly. **S**tressors, **t**oxins, **a**llergens, **m**icrobes, and **p**oor diet contribute, but the preceding emotional conflicts are the spark. Biological Decoding illuminates these hidden origins.

Challenges, both internal and external, are often tied to rigid thought patterns and unresolved emotional burdens. Clinging to perspectives without curiosity sustains disease. This book shows how unresolved psychological energy manifests physically, offering a roadmap for self-awareness and true healing.

The history of science is not a linear progression, but rather a series of paradigm shifts. Much like Planck's revolution in physics, this book steps beyond traditional medicine to show how beliefs can be the architects of disease.

RABBIT HOLE

Dr. Eben Alexander III, Neurosurgeon – *The Proof of Heaven*

CHAPTER 3

REDEFINING NORMAL:
REMOVE THE "CRAZY PERSON" LABEL

I grew up in the 80s.

This was an era of thought in which talking about mental health was forbidden within families. Mine was no different. My mother struggled with what appeared to us as significant emotional and mental health challenges that resulted in behaviors that most would see, even today, as 'crazy.' I have many childhood memories of my mom and how her mental health ravaged her and my dad, and how it shaped the kind of physician I am today. I share this not to disparage my mom but to remind each of you that the inner world of our thoughts is the riddle and key to aligning our mental and physical health with our already perfect spirit.

A simple road trip could turn into a 48-hour nightmare because of a misplaced shadow. My mom, whose fear of flying kept us on the ground, had a mind to conjure catastrophe from inanimate objects. If she saw something on the side of the road, anything bigger than a milk carton, her sense of reality would sometimes disconnect from what the rest of us were perceiving. That object would become a baby in her mind. In her convinced certainty, my dad had just run over it and killed it. We would hold our breath, knowing that once this thought took root, our vacation was over. For us, road trips weren't a family adventure, but a test of our endurance, waiting for the inevitable chaos to arrive.

My mom was a very loving and doting mother in many ways, but specific triggers would set her off and unleash absolute chaos for everyone. During those episodes, she could become intensely distressed, sometimes crying, yelling, or physically reacting in ways that were extremely hard on my father and all of us. Sometimes, she'd try to grab the steering wheel, forcing me to hold her down while my dad searched for a safe place to stop. Once we found a hotel, my dad would spend hours, sometimes 12 or more, calming her down. Eventually, her overactive mind would exhaust her, and she'd sleep for 18 hours or more. When she woke up, it was as if nothing had happened; her mind had reset entirely.

Meanwhile, my dad, emotionally drained and physically worn, carried the invisible scars of what had unfolded. As a family, we fell into an unspoken agreement to pretend everything was normal. We wouldn't talk about any of it - the fear, the irrationality, we just swept it all under the proverbial rug and went about our vacation.

This is just scratching the surface of my experience as a child navigating mental health challenges within my family. While my sisters saw it as a nuisance or something strange to be avoided, I approached it differently. I wanted to understand it, to figure out why it was happening. By the time things reached their peak, my sisters had already moved on to college and beyond, leaving my dad and me to manage my mom's struggles alone. We tried everything we could think of to help her.

One of our more elaborate attempts involved using one of those massive 1980s camcorders to film the garbage we found along the side of the roads. We would drive up to the trash, show her the footage, and even get out of the car and pick it up while recording, hoping she could watch these videos later, in the comfort of her home. Our logic was that seeing the garbage on film might prove to her how her mind was playing tricks on her, teaching her brain to think differently moving forward. It was just one of the many creative things we tried, but none made a difference. Applying logic to irrationality would never work.

What I learned, repeatedly as a young person, was that emotional responses aren't driven by logic. No matter how much reason we brought to the table, it couldn't touch the depth of what my mom was experiencing. That realization shaped the way I understood both her and the unpredictable nature of mental health, and later, I came to appreciate that it's our subconscious programming that is truly in the driver's seat.

My dad, a practicing Ear, Nose, Throat, and Facial Plastic Surgeon, lacked significant training in psychiatry. Over the years, my mom regularly saw many psychiatrists and therapists, yet their efforts seemed futile. Her breakdowns became so predictable that my dad and I began preparing the backseat of our car as a makeshift bed, encouraging her to lie down so that we could go on a road trip and avoid what felt like irrational triggers.

In 1988, Prozac, the very first SSRI, was introduced. Say what you will about antidepressants, but this drug profoundly changed the lives of my mom and my dad. When I entered college in 1990, I remember calling my dad near the end of my first year to ask how Mom was doing during car rides. Hesitantly, as if not wanting to jinx it, he told me it had been nearly a year since her last episode. At the peak of her condition, my poor mom was prescribed 160mg daily, far above the typical 20-40mg dosage, costing my dad almost $400 a month, which is equivalent to nearly $1,000 today. Today, Prozac costs as little as a $5 co-pay, but I vividly recall my dad saying he would pay ten times that amount for the peace it brought them.

For my parents, Prozac was a kind of miracle. As empty nesters, they could finally travel and enjoy a calm that had once seemed so out of reach. But miracles often come at a price. Watching my mom over the years, and hundreds of patients since, has shown me that unreleased harmful emotional conflicts carry an invisible yet substantial cost. It is the inspiration for my writing this book. My mom, who is still alive, continues to pay that price to this day.

The introduction of Prozac marked a massive breakthrough in psychiatric care, giving rise to a new era of medications and our understanding of the brain's biochemical signals called neurotransmitters. But this breakthrough also bred complacency. We stopped asking questions and innovating in this area of medical psychiatry. Greed took over the pharmaceutical industry. Following the profit model, Big Pharma began focusing on rebranding strategies rather than innovation, repurposing SSRIs for a growing list of conditions: anxiety, depression, OCD, PTSD, premenstrual dysphoric disorder (PMDD), hot flashes, bulimia, irritable bowel syndrome, and even pain.

I can speak on this with authority because I believed in it wholeheartedly; I drank the Kool-Aid. Prozac's success with my mom convinced me it was a gift from above, and I prescribed it to countless patients struggling with mental illness. I even took it for years myself. It aligned with the prevailing medical belief that mental health issues stem from biochemical imbalances. But as I later realized, the root causes often get unconsciously suppressed. My parents' story is just one among millions.

For years, my mom's outbursts subsided, and my parents stopped searching for the root cause of her illness since it was being managed. My mom has now taken Prozac religiously ever since. By her late 70s, she started driving again after nearly 40 years. From the outside, it looked like a triumph. But as her son, as a physician, I see it differently. It came with a slow death knell.

I support the use of medications like Prozac in appropriate situations. These medications can serve as a bridge, a tool helping people like my mom confront the emotional conflicts that initially led to her mental breakdowns. However, hindsight is 20/20. Years later, having heard more of my mom's stories, especially those from the year before her first episode, it became clearer to me what contributed to her early breakdowns. Yet, she and my dad, like many others, focused on the major victory and stopped asking the most important question we can ask about any disease or dysfunction: Why did this happen in the first place? What is the origin story? By neglecting to explore that, my mom paid a heavy price.

Over the decades, I have seen the toll SSRIs can take, especially on women. For many, these medications significantly affect libido, which can strain even the healthiest marriages. However, this is not the cost I am referring to. The hidden cost is far greater. Today, my mom, in her mid-80s, feels very different from the vibrant woman I remember growing up with, and it saddens me to see how emotionally withdrawn and exhausted she often seems. She struggles to process any negative emotions and has lost much of her empathy for others. When life becomes overwhelming, which happens often, she retreats into sleep. My father, in many ways, has become her emotional caretaker, acting almost like a surrogate parent. My mom stopped seeking new experiences or knowledge decades ago, having lost the desire to learn anything new; she isn't curious about much of anything anymore. She has become an NPC (Non-Player Character) at Earth School. More on that later.

Looking back, it's clear Prozac helped suppress the chaos, but it never tackled the root cause. My mom's unresolved emotional conflicts, which form the foundation of her struggles, were left unexplored, and she had some traumas that needed attention. While Prozac provided chemical stability, it also significantly hindered her growth. For my mother, it seemed over time to blunt her emotional range which is the fuel for creativity, thought, and the desire for new experiences. This means that she never fully addressed her emotional issues. One way she allowed this to manifest was in her relationships with her family. It caused a rift with her grandchildren, who grew distant and showed disrespect because of her lack of connection and curiosity about their lives.

Physically, her unprocessed emotional conflicts contributed to later health problems as she suffered from POTS (Positional Orthostatic Tachycardia Syndrome), which causes your blood pressure to drop, so you have to lie down. She dealt with her emotions best when she lay in bed, so her body created a way to ensure that. In the year prior to my mom's stroke, I decided to stop communicating with my father. His growing hate towards me (more on that later) was so palpable that I felt it in my mind, emotions, and body, which also impacted my own family. In retaliation, my dad shared things about me that I believed were untrue and deeply hurtful and my mom would, in turn, not talk to me.

Although I showed my mom evidence that contradicted what my dad said, she understandably wanted to maintain peace with my dad. Whenever she tried to talk to him and defend me, my father would shut her down. Within a year of this, my mother had a stroke that affected the part of her brain primarily responsible for her speech.

Through the lens of Biological Decoding—an interpretive framework I explore in this book—strokes are sometimes symbolically associated with unresolved emotional conflicts or perceived losses of connection. I don't present this as proven medical fact, but as one of several lenses through which I've tried to understand what happened. Today, my dad blames me for my mom's stroke. While I can confidently say that it was related to the conflict between us, it was also due to her inability to process her emotions properly, as you'll soon learn in even greater detail.

My mom truly embodied love when I was growing up, yet her emotional landscape was ravaged over the years by unresolved conflicts that were never weeded out. Every family has stories of conflict and my mom's story is just one of many that demonstrate how biological dysfunction, also known as disease, can take hold when those emotional landscapes aren't cleared out to make way for healing.

Prozac, like most medications, should not be thought of as filling a deficiency indefinitely. We are not Prozac deficient, just as we are not deficient in statins, blood pressure medications, or antacids. Our bodies are exquisitely designed, and when they stop functioning as we expect, I would urge us to start recognizing that it could be because our bodies are creating a new physical design to symbolically represent our unconsciously unreleased emotional conflicts. This is not pseudoscience. This is how epigenetics influences biology through gene expression, as dictated by the signals transmitted. Is more confirmatory science required? Absolutely. But connecting the dots is my life's mission. Opening your mind to a new thought paradigm is my purpose, my "one-thing."

What my mom sadly experienced was often dismissed as "crazy," a word that has become a ubiquitous label today. But calling someone "crazy" is lazy, dismissive, and intolerant. It reflects our unwillingness to ask more profound questions. We must move beyond these superficial judgments and labels to better understand ourselves and others and to become curious observers.

Thoughts are the architects of our beliefs and behaviors, intricately connected to our emotions. However, rigid thoughts lead to rigid emotions. As humans, we experience a range of emotions that are far more nuanced than those of animals. Brené Brown, a well-known author and social science scholar, has identified 87 distinct emotions. To make it simpler, I'll start with the eight primary emotions: happiness, sadness, trust, fear, surprise, anticipation, anger, and disgust. Navigating these emotions is like finding the right lens at the optometrist, bringing clarity to the discordance within.

RABBIT HOLE
Dr. Bruce Lipton - *The Biology of Belief*

CHAPTER 4

TAKING A C.A.B. RIDE
WITH YOUR THOUGHTS

The best version of any person emerges, not from medication or a flawless diet, but from a creative act that begins in the mind. Wellness starts with your thoughts, and when they are filled with love, joy, and gratitude, they become the fabric for vibrant, self-sustaining health. These powerful, positive emotions give rise to three essential elements that align our humanity and physicality at their highest level.

This process is a fundamental skill that can be developed and strengthened. I call it taking **the C.A.B ride** with your emotional thoughts:

- **C**uriosity: about the thought behind your emotion
- **A**wareness: of the precise emotion and where you feel it in your body
- **B**oomerang: that energy in a way that creates positivity and redirects your focus

Unfortunately, in my mom's case, her belief system was shaped by unresolved emotional conflicts that persisted for decades, fueling negative feelings like fear and helplessness. Instead of fostering connection and growth, these emotions took a different **C.A.B. ride:** one lacking **C**uriosity, **A**wareness, and consciousness of its **B**oomerang effect.

The result was a loss of emotional bonds with her grandchildren, a decreased understanding of her inner world, and a limited capacity to give and receive love. This emotional distance unintentionally boomeranged back as apathy from others, reflecting what she unconsciously projected. The emotions we receive from others, whether positive or negative, are often earned based on whether our **C.A.B.** aligns with or conflicts with our core beliefs. Ultimately, how we choose to guide our own **C.A.B.** with each thought determines whether we nurture health or dysfunction in our lives.

The Student of Earth School

Imagine you're from another planet and have been assigned to Earth School to study the peculiar species known as humans. Your mission is to understand their biology, environments, and collective behaviors. As you observe, patterns begin to emerge: shared perceptions, beliefs, and obstacles that shape human consciousness. You'd learn how biology influences choices, how sensations steer decisions, and how those forces affect longevity and well-being.

Depending on how these consciousnesses dance together, you'd also see how each person's conflicts, shaped by parents, siblings, and life experience, can lead to either suffering or growth.

In the 25-plus years I've been practicing medicine, I've been honored to listen to countless stories, each offering a window into the emotional lives of my patients. As a medical student I learned the fundamentals of science and medicine through rigorous study and by absorbing objective, observable facts. During my final two years of medical school, I shadowed physicians across various specialties and began to notice recurring patterns in how physical diseases presented. Residency sharpened my focus, immersing me in a specialty while also revealing blind spots in my thinking. Those gaps widened as my experience grew, and I could no longer ignore them. As much as formal training built my foundation, the stories of my patients have been my truest education, my "Earth School." I've noticed a recurring truth: while external forces like **S.T.A.M.P. triggers** can threaten <u>physical</u> health, few things shape our well-being as powerfully as what we believe.

Every illness and every state of wellness starts with a thought.

A single idea of unworthiness, for example, can trigger a surge of stress hormones, impair immune function, and ultimately lead to biological changes that we come to recognize as disease. Thoughts shape emotions, which then affect behavior, biochemistry, neural pathways, hormone responses, and even gene expression. This is **the C.A.B. ride** of emotional thoughts, a journey that ties directly to the core idea behind Biological Decoding.

There Is No Graduation Date from Earth School

This journey mirrors life itself.

We must undertake the **C.A.B. ride** of self-discovery with our thoughts to grow as individuals. Let curiosity about ourselves, our awareness, the emotions our thoughts evoke, and the willingness to send that energy outward expansively to become a part of our daily existence. Along the way, we must identify the blind spots in our thinking and replace them with higher paradigms that uplift our health, relationships, and overall sense of purpose, extending to those around us.

Even now, over 25 years into my medical career, I remain a student at Earth School. Every day offers a new lesson about what it means to be a healthy and whole human. People often speak of "enlightenment" as an endpoint, but no accurate graduation date exists. Understanding ourselves, thoughts, emotions, and creative capacity is an ongoing journey. This journey only deepens and becomes more rewarding and profound over time.

RABBIT HOLE

Dr. Michael Newton, psychiatrist, author and hypnotherapist

– *The Journey of Souls*

CHAPTER 5

THE GAME OF LIFE: LESSONS FROM EARTH SCHOOL

Earth School is not an exclusive institution; it is open to everyone. It requires no special qualifications, just a willingness to explore, learn, and, most importantly, grow. I invite you to see yourself as a fellow student, exploring the depths of your being, trusting your instincts, and gradually gaining wisdom by recognizing your blind spots. With humility, acknowledge that there's always more to learn. By sharpening your perception, increasing your awareness, and broadening your perspective, you can navigate the stages of life with greater ease and grace.

I've never been much of a gamer. I grew up in the age of Donkey Kong and Pac-Man. I dabbled in Street Fighter but never found much lasting joy in video games. I channeled my energy into competitive sports, which offered me a different perspective: Life is a game.

When I call life a game, I don't mean one of manipulation or deceit. I'm referring to a game with evolving rules, shaped by the legal system, societal norms, and moral codes. These rules are constantly in flux, influenced by age, geography, social status, and the evolving generational mindsets that collectively shape human consciousness. Our greatest strength as humans lies in our ability to adapt, to transform, and thrive in the face of change.

Reflect on the rapid technological and social changes you've witnessed, especially if you grew up before the 1990s or earlier. These shifts have demanded a great deal of adaptability. Recall a time when restaurants had cigarette machines and were divided into "smoking" and "non-smoking" sections. That was typical in the 1980s. Now, that concept feels outdated, as if it disappeared overnight.

Navigation tells a similar story. Paper maps were tucked away in every car's glove compartment not long ago. Then came stand-alone GPS devices. Now, smartphones provide turn-by-turn directions, and self-driving vehicles are gaining traction. What once seemed unimaginable has become a part of our everyday reality, known as the human consciousness.

The thought archetypes we live by today were mere fantasy in the past. Our assumptions about what's possible are often invisible to us until we stop and question them. My aim for you is to start doing just that: challenge the assumptions you hold unconsciously, ask how you arrived at this point, and consider how things could be different. By questioning these assumptions, you can open the door to new possibilities and embrace the potential for positive change.

Lessons from the Unexpected

Let's ground this concept in recent history. Imagine that before 2020, someone told you the following would happen within two hours:

- Tom Hanks, in Australia, would be the first celebrity diagnosed with a novel coronavirus

- The NBA would suddenly suspend its season.

- The President of the United States would put a ground stop on all international flights into the U.S.

These events, taken together, would have sounded absurd. Yet in 2020, they unfolded in real time, reshaping our lives overnight.

Or think about cultural shifts:

- The name "Karen" has become a meme for entitled behavior, and it is now being used as a verb.

- Coffee shops where people once read newspapers are now filled with people quietly scrolling on their phones instead.

- You watch a DIY video on your phone, tap a few buttons, and the featured product is delivered to your doorstep in less than 24 hours.

These examples show how the thought archetypes of the past often shape every aspect of today's world without our conscious awareness.

Embracing the Role of a Student of Earth School

When you accept your role as a student in Earth School, you begin to see Life as an ongoing discovery process. You notice the subtle shifts in the game, observing your thoughts about the collective human consciousness. This awareness empowers you to live with more love, peace, and curiosity. Most importantly, you develop thought flexibility - the ability to adapt your thinking as the game's rules evolve.

There's a reason older generations sometimes struggle with the ways of younger generations: they hold firmly to the thought patterns of their youth, resisting the new paradigms of today. But true wisdom lies in embracing both. The lessons of the past and the possibilities of the future are keys to growth, and the bridge between is maintaining curiosity and openness.

I've observed a powerful pattern in my work with patients across the generational spectrum, including those in end-of-life care scenarios. Those who find peace in their later years are the ones who hold space for both the wisdom of their youth and the evolving perspectives of younger generations. They approach their final days as a gift, not something to be feared or resisted.

RABBIT HOLE
Dolores Cannon – "Past Life Regression Hypnotherapy"

CHAPTER 6

LIVING IN THE GREY: FINDING FREEDOM BEYOND BLACK-AND-WHITE THINKING

From as early as I can remember, my dad and I clashed on nearly every major topic.

He believed every idea had a clear-cut answer: right or wrong, fact or fallacy. To him, being "loosey-goosey" with your thoughts meant you were part of the problem, and not taking a firm stance was an unforgivable offense. "If you don't pick a side," he'd say, "no one will know where you stand, and neither will you." His thinking was as concrete and black-and-white as you could get. He treated everything like a **zero-sum game**.

Growing up, those words bothered me. They made me feel like my way of thinking was wrong, influencing how I saw the world. I didn't fully align with either political extreme. But in his eyes, not being a Republican automatically made me a Democrat, and if I wasn't one or the other, I felt defective and I lacked clarity in my thoughts. My principles and values seemed invalidated by his perfectly-formed conclusions.

This black-and-white thinking led to endless debates that always seemed to end with one winner: my dad.

Whether we argued about gay rights, obesity, early views on HIV, religion, or education, he allowed no middle ground, no space for uncertainty. Even personal questions, like the nature vs. nurture debate surrounding my oldest adopted sister, became battlegrounds. Every discussion felt like a zero-sum game he had to win. **His unwavering certainty left little room for curiosity, empathy, or alternative perspectives**. The most exhausting part wasn't the arguments themselves, but the steady erosion of feeling heard, each attempt at understanding met with dismissal.

Looking back, it's almost amusing how much we managed to irritate each other.

Where he saw absolutes, I saw nuance; where he demanded certainty, I leaned into curiosity. Most issues I believed lived in the messy in-between, what I call grey thinking, while he insisted on drawing hard lines in the sand. This fundamental difference didn't just fuel our debates, it defined our relationship.

Over time, it created a chasm: he came to view me not only as a disappointment but also as a threat to his worldview. That judgment still stings, but it also sharpened my commitment to questioning assumptions, embracing complexity, and searching for truth outside rigid binaries. The very friction that distanced us also shaped who I became.

It wasn't until my third midlife crisis (yes, my third) that I finally stopped letting his judgment shape me.

The Three Crises

My first midlife crisis came in my early 30s when I stepped away from Catholicism in search of something beyond its traditions. Please don't misunderstand me - I deeply cherished my Catholic upbringing and the richness of its rituals. For years, it gave me a deep sense of peace...until one day, it didn't. The resonance I once felt simply faded.

This shift was a genuine crisis. I had gone to Catholic schools from first grade through college. Every girlfriend and close friend up until medical school was Catholic. And my father, the man I had placed on the highest pedestal, was the most devoted Catholic I knew. Walking away felt like abandoning not only my faith but also the people in it, especially him. When I finally told my father, he didn't speak to me for two years.

My second crisis, this one lining up more accurately with the phrase "midlife crisis," arrived in my early 40s, when I turned toward Functional Medicine. Like the first, I felt I was betraying everything I had learned up to that point. It felt like an exile from the very community of teachers, mentors, and colleagues who had trained me.

The third crisis hit in my early 50s (my wife hopes it's the last, ha!). I call this one my "Life Sabbatical." It was a two-year deep dive into my mortality, beliefs, and the choices I had made up to this juncture in my life. Unlike earlier crises, which carried a sense of betraying a collective (religion or medicine), this one was personal. I was holding up a mirror to myself.

Without fully realizing it at first, I confronted every emotional trigger in my life, one by one. I took an arborist's approach to my inner landscape—trimming, pruning, and pulling out the weeds of my subconscious. Through this process, I found clarity about who I truly was. I decided I would no longer carry fear, shame, guilt, or the weight of comparison. I became far more emotionally regulated, strengthening the most crucial relationship in my life: my marriage.

Shifting my thought paradigms left lasting impressions and lessons.

It was messy, disorienting, and beautiful. With each of my three crises, I was leaving behind the 'old' and embracing the 'new.' New can feel like betrayal to yourself and others, but each time I followed my heart's energy and intuition, it proved to be an accurate life compass.

Yet, the lesson I also learned from each pivot was that these experiences were about honoring the most powerful principle in life: change is inevitable. It was not about abandonment or betrayal, but rather about my **collaborative story** - that without one part, the others made less sense. If I did not listen to the deepest parts of me, I would naturally hit larger, much more destructive walls until I learned to listen and evolve. As the saying goes: "What we resist, persists."

Humans have an extraordinary capacity to evolve, create, and heal.

That journey starts with flexible, grey thinking and the willingness to challenge not only others' beliefs, but also our own. We do that by asking the difficult questions: are my beliefs truly mine? Or are they ones downloaded into my hardware?

Still unsure where to start with this?

Start with any topic or word that creates a deep emotional response, especially a dysregulated one. This is your entry point. Do you already feel regulated? Then move to the beliefs you hold to so firmly you think everyone else is wrong—beliefs that, perhaps, tend to trigger others. (These could be your beliefs, gift-wrapped in selfishness. Those require an even deeper plunge.)

It is important to understand that everyone has these firmly-held beliefs, even the ones in wrapped with a tinge of narcissism. My reminder to you is this: the more uncomfortable it makes you feel, the more assured you can be that you're going in the right direction. Your ego will try to keep you from taking this journey, but as I was often reminded by some wise people as I went through my crises: "walk through the fire and not around it because on the other side lies peace."

Rigid Thinking and Its Biological Impact

For the first half of my medical career, I relied almost exclusively on science since the modeling of my father, also a physician, suggested that if I dared to dabble even slightly on the fringes of thought, I would be met with shame or guilt from the medical community. Anything "hippy-dippy," as my dad would say, seemed absurd. Therefore, for a time, I limited myself to what I could observe with my five senses.

Today, neuroscientists like Dr. Tara Swart note that we have over 30 senses that we've yet to fully tap into. Additionally, I have found that embracing my more natural inclination toward grey thinking, even in medicine, has liberated me and allowed me to meaningfully alter my patients' health trajectories based on their stories, not simply my own limited lens.

Rigid thought paradigms, by design, block creativity, harm relationships, weaken inner peace, and limit healing in all areas of life. Negative emotions like shame, guilt, and fear intensify signals through the body, influencing gene expression and the blueprint of our health. In my case, ankylosing spondylitis arose as my genes responded to chronic emotional stress and unresolved internal conflict, a tension between supporting my father emotionally and reconciling his rigid worldview versus honoring my authentic self and my own belief system that honored grey thinking.

Here's where epigenetics comes in.

Genes don't act alone. Your body doesn't make decisions randomly. Your genes respond to signals, which include signals from your environment in additional to all the signals your body relays—like the ones that originate from your beliefs which shape your emotional state and your perception of stressors. This isn't abstract philosophy; it's the embodiment of biology in real-time.

Genes as Copy Machines

Here's the simplified version: genes are blueprints. They tell your cells how to build proteins—the building blocks of every tissue, organ, and function in your body. But here's the twist: before that "blueprint" is transcribed into a protein, it gets run through a process called **post-transcriptional modification**, like an editing bay for your DNA.

Think of a gene like a copy machine. You expect it to make an exact copy of whatever you place on the glass. But before the copy is made, it undergoes edits, small tweaks or major changes, based on the signals that your cell membrane received and transmitted to your genes. So, the final protein might be vastly different from the original "blueprint" copy. In fact, a single gene can produce *hundreds* of other proteins.

The Paradox of Evidence-Based Medicine

Evidence-based medicine is invaluable, but the human body isn't a machine. It's a symphony of interconnected signals. Even the best studies can't account for everything. That's why I combine rigorous data, obtained through studies called meta-analyses, with intuition. Wisdom isn't about clinging to facts; it's about discerning which facts matter and remaining open to new ones.

Consider hormone replacement therapy (HRT) for postmenopausal women. A 2002 study showed increased risks of heart disease and breast cancer. As a result, HRT use dropped 46% in the US over the following year. However, women who stopped HRT experienced hot flashes, sleep issues, mood swings, vaginal dryness, accelerated bone loss, and more.

Traditional medical physicians who hold onto the findings of this original study persistently push back requests to help their female patients with HRT. Personalized medicine today embraces grey thinking, recognizing that later studies revealed that timing, delivery method, and the type of progesterone dramatically affected outcomes. Avoiding a rare heart risk inadvertently exposed thousands to greater harm, like hip fractures, which carry a higher mortality rate within the first year than heart attacks.

Science, like life, exists in the grey. Facts are relative, context-dependent, and subject to evolution. A single study shouldn't dictate absolute truths. Yet, physicians love to quote a particular study for or against a particular therapy overlooking that health outcomes must be personalized.

Living in the Grey: History and Physics

History is replete with examples where rigid thinking hindered progress. Galileo challenged the Catholic Church by asserting the Earth revolved around the Sun, a statement that was considered dangerous, even life-threatening. Paradigms only shift when someone dares to ask: **What if we have been seeing it all wrong?**

Quantum physicists like Niels Bohr, Max Planck, and Albert Einstein embraced uncertainty, exploring the unseen through mathematics, intuition, and curiosity. They proved that growth flourishes in the grey. Science demands measurable evidence, yet simultaneously acknowledges invisible forces, like light waves or sound frequencies. Grey thinking exists in this tension between the seen and the unseen.

Case in Point: George Washington

George Washington, America's first president, died at age 68. The day before he got sick, he rode on horseback through a snowy Mount Vernon and stayed in his wet clothes to avoid being late for dinner. The next day, he had a sore throat. But he pushed through, working outdoors anyway.

Two days later, still sick, he called for help. Back then, illness was believed to stem from "bad blood," so the standard treatment was, you guessed it, bloodletting. His secretary, Albin Rawlins, bled him. Doctors came and bled him four more times over eight hours, removing 40% of his blood.

Washington's doctors didn't just fail him, they likely killed him. Not because they were malicious, but because their *thought paradigm*, their belief in bloodletting, was flawed.

Today, we know Washington likely had bacterial pertussis, easily treatable with modern antibiotics. But if I had traveled back in time with a Z-pack and offered it, Washington might've called for my arrest. Germ theory didn't exist yet. Antibiotics weren't even imagined.

That's the power, and the danger, of rigid thinking. Paradigms shape perception. What seems "impossible" today may become an obvious truth tomorrow.

The Gluten Lesson

I once dismissed gluten-free diets for non-celiac patients as "crazy," ignoring patients' stories and intuition. By 2006, research revealed gluten influences Zonulin, increasing intestinal permeability even in non-celiac individuals. Molecular mimicry explained links between gluten and autoimmune thyroid disease. My early, rigid thinking delayed adopting these insights, limiting care to countless patients.

As a professional, I learned that grey thinking necessitates taking **a C.A.B ride (C**uriosity, **A**wareness, **B**oomerang) with my beliefs in order to expand my lenses and help more patients. It also allows for the integration of evidence with intuition as my co-pilot.

Consider diet debates, such as vegan versus carnivore. These often devolve into rigid ideologies. But the truth is more nuanced: our choices are shaped by culture, religion, family, life experiences, and even the unique tolerances of our own GI tract. Judging others without understanding their stories robs us of connection and in my world, the opportunity to help them heal. **Living in the grey means holding space for the idea that multiple possibilities can exist simultaneously—this is quantum thinking**. This mindset eases the tension between our own beliefs and the beliefs of others, reducing the negative emotional triggers that ultimately harm both our health and our biology.

The Takeaway: You Are Always Becoming

Your thoughts, beliefs, and emotions send signals to your genes, shaping how the next version of yourself emerges. Thinking in grey, releasing rigid beliefs, and embracing uncertainty keep you curious and open the door to positively influencing your biology. This is biological decoding at its core; every cellular protein your body produces reflects the conflicts between your own beliefs and those imposed by the world around you.

What signals are you sending?

Will your future self be guided by ego? Or will you be free of it, in a place where emotional regulation thrives, creating an inner peace untouched by the disease of limiting beliefs? This does not mean you will not feel emotions, but you will live with the knowledge that everything will be okay, actively participating in the evolution of your optimal self.

RABBIT HOLE
Quantum Field Theory

CHAPTER 7

ENERGY: THE GREY FORCE OF LIFE

Let's dive into quantum physics, keeping in mind that energy isn't just a concept from physics - it is the very foundation of our makeup. Don't worry, I won't get lost in complex equations or linear algebra, since I am no mathematician, and you don't need to be either. However, understanding the basics is crucial because without this foundation, energy medicine and Biological Decoding can easily be dismissed as fringe ideas, rather than recognized as deeply grounded, scientifically informed approaches.

Science today agrees that everything, including you, is inseparable from energy. Einstein gave us the shorthand in his famous equation:

$$E = mc^2$$

M is mass, the "stuff" that makes up matter, and c is the speed of light. We all recognize this formula, but few pause to grasp its meaning and how it applies in our everyday lives.

Analogy: The Battery – Potential Energy

Think of mass like a giant battery sitting on a shelf. All the energy is in there, stored and waiting, but you can't use it to power anything until you connect it to a circuit. Once it's released, though, the energy becomes usable. Einstein showed us that mass is just this kind of stored energy, and c^2 —the speed of light squared — is the enormous conversion factor, like flipping a tiny switch that unleashes a massive current. Think of nuclear reactions to appreciate the enormous energy that can be released.

How This Ties into Quantum Physics

If Einstein gave us the big picture, quantum physics zooms into the fine print. At everyday scales, your desk, your phone, your body seem solid. But zoom in, and everything turns into a buzzing dance between matter and energy. Mass is like a tightly coiled spring at the quantum level. To the naked eye, it looks still and solid. But quantum physics shows us that it's full of invisible motion and binding forces. The equation tells us just how much potential is wound up in that spring. Unlock it, and you don't just release a little energy, you unleash a staggering amount because c2 is such a huge multiplier.

This brings us to **Quantum Field Theory (QFT)**, the modern foundation of physics. While Einstein revealed the link between mass and energy, QFT explains how they behave. It tells us the universe is built from fields, and particles are simply ripples or excitations in those fields, like waves rising from the surface of the ocean. Everything we see, including our own bodies, emerges from this invisible ocean. In that sense, energy isn't only the currency of matter, it's the fabric of reality itself.

Looking Closer: What Is Matter Made Of?

In school, we learned that cells are the building blocks of life.

Then we discovered that cells are made of molecules, and molecules are made up of atoms. For a long time, atoms were thought to be indivisible. It reminds me of the funny dad joke: "Why can't you trust an atom? Because they make up everything!"

But science, driven by "grey thinkers" unwilling to stop asking questions, dug deeper. Atoms were made up of protons, neutrons, and electrons. Further questioning of this "truth" revealed that protons and neutrons were composed of even smaller particles called quarks. A proton is two "up" quarks and one "down." A neutron is two "down" quarks and one "up." Think of quarks as Lego bricks, the pieces behind the pieces.

The Large Hadron Collider: Crashing Reality Apart

You can't just put a quark under a microscope.

To discover them, physicists built the **Large Hadron Collider**, a 17-mile underground ring in Europe where protons are accelerated close to the speed of light and smashed together. It's Earth's biggest demolition derby. But instead of twisted metal, the wreckage reveals quarks, gluons, and stranger particles.

Experiments like these confirmed that quarks exist, gluons hold them together, and most famously, the **Higgs boson** was discovered. The Higgs field explains why particles have mass at all. Without it, nothing would clump together, no stars, no planets, no you.

In other words, this isn't abstract science; it's the reason matter exists at all. The fact that physicists can recreate, study, and confirm these individual building blocks reminds us that our very existence depends on laws of nature far stranger than classical physics had us believing. It is also a reminder of the limitations of using only our senses as truth and fact.

Wave and Particle, Just Like Us

Here's where things get really fascinating.

Subatomic particles don't behave like everyday objects. Sometimes they act like particles, sometimes like waves. The Quantum Field Theory shows us that wave and particle are two sides of the same coin. At the smallest scales, the universe isn't solid but a fluctuating field of probabilities, a canvas of all possibilities. Each particle has its own unique field within a larger unifying field. Basically, fields influence and interact with each other.

And this isn't so different from our inner world.

Thoughts and emotions don't behave like fixed objects either. They ebb, flow, collide, and ripple outward, more like waves. Matter itself is mostly space dotted with energetic ripples. If you stripped a box of every particle, what remains wouldn't be "nothing" but a sea of frequencies still humming in motion.

Why This Matters for Medicine and Biological Decoding

Quantum physics underpins everything. It teaches us that everything is connected to energy: adaptable, ever-changing, and constantly interacting. When energies collide, they ripple outward like stones thrown into a pond. They can attract, repel, distort, or align. Though invisible, their effects are undeniable.

Here's the revelation: **thought is energy, emotion is energy, and you yourself are composed of energy.** And energy is never static.

It vibrates in frequencies and amplitudes, always in motion. We see this in simple ways: a low bass note can rattle a windowpane, while a high-pitched violin string can move us to tears. The difference isn't the existence of energy, but the frequency it carries.

Human beings are no different; our thoughts and emotions generate patterns that ripple outwards, interacting with others and shaping the environments we inhabit. Once I grasped that everything —yes, everything— is woven from the same energetic field fabric described by physics, it transformed how I practiced medicine and how I lived my life. The boundaries between "me" and "you" are far less real than they appear. We are participants in a single, unified energetic field, resonating with and influencing one another in ways we are only beginning to understand, which also impacts our biology.

Picture this:

You are at a crowded party and across the room, your best friend walks in. Before you see their face, you feel their presence; your body relaxes, your mood lifts. Now imagine the opposite: someone you've had a conflict with enters, and you sense tension before a word is spoken. That "energy shift" isn't mystical; it's resonance.

Our bodies are constantly reading subtle cues: facial expressions, posture, tone, and even electrical fields generated by the heart and brain. These interactions change our internal frequency, triggering chemical cascades that influence stress hormones, immunity, and even gene expression. In this way, thoughts and emotions aren't abstract; they ripple through your biology, shaping health or disease. In the spirit of Dr. Joe Dispenza, "Would you agree that if a negative belief can make you ill, then a positive belief can make you heal?" It does at least offer pause when it comes to the quality of our thoughts.

Rigid, negative thoughts combined with strong emotions generate powerful energetic waves that can alter biology and even gene expression. Over time, this may manifest as illness. Conversely, flexible thinking expands your inner pond into something more like an ocean, able to absorb disruptions without tipping into chaos.

The Energy Aware Conductor: A Harmonious Symphony

Imagine your body as an orchestra led by a wise conductor.

The strings (emotions) play melodies that rise and fall, shaping the overall tone of your internal energy. The winds (your neuroendocrine system) carry the tune forward with feel-good hormones like serotonin, dopamine, and oxytocin. The percussion (your immune system) keeps the steady rhythm, defending against threats without drowning out the music. And the brass (genes) respond dynamically, activating healing, repair, and resilience in sync with the score.

Like any orchestra, the key lies in frequency and resonance. When the conductor (your mind) is grounded in curiosity, gratitude, and openness, each section plays in tune, creating harmony. That harmony is a frequency your whole body resonates with, rippling outwards into your relationships and environment. But when the conductor is overwhelmed by fear, anger, or rigidity, the sections fall out of sync, producing dissonance as stress hormones surge, immune rhythms falter, and genes switch into defense mode. Over time, that dissonance shapes disease, just as harmony fosters healing. In other words, your inner frequency doesn't just influence how you feel; it orchestrates your biology and the energy you share with the world.

To understand how sound influences our biology and energy, we can look to the Solfeggio frequencies—specific tones believed to naturally resonate with different parts of the body, supporting balance, healing, and coherence. Instruments such as singing bowls, gongs, and tuning forks create vibrations that the body readily responds to.

Low-frequency gongs (30-60 Hz) penetrate the chest and diaphragm, encouraging deep breathing, lymphatic flow, and healthy circulation. Higher-frequency bowls (400-1000 Hz) resonate more with the cranial cavity, sinuses, and throat, often promoting mental clarity and nervous system balance. Certain frequencies, like 528 Hz, are even associated with cellular repair and overall energetic harmony.

These vibrations can entrain brainwaves, slow the heart rate, and balance the nervous system—helping to create coherence throughout the body. In this way, sound doesn't just touch the surface; it actively shifts internal energy patterns, influencing hormone levels, immune function, and even gene expression.

Just as with our thoughts and emotions, sound demonstrates a universal principle: energy in motion shapes the body, guiding it toward balance and healing.

Why talk about energy at all?

Humans have always wrestled with three central questions:

1. Where did I come from?

2. What is my purpose?

3. Why did I get this disease? (the essence of this book)

Understanding energy begins to connect these.

Thoughts create emotions, which drive behaviors, which in turn shift our chemistry and nervous system, ultimately directing hormones, cells, and genes. Rigid beliefs in thinking program the body to work within a narrower range of options. A flexible energy of thought opens us up to all possibilities for healing which is the field that embraces everything that our quantum physicist's friends have taught.

Curiosity is what drives progress.

The most vital journey isn't outward, but inward—becoming students of ourselves. It isn't about obsessing over why others act as they do, but holding up the mirror and asking those questions of ourselves. The people who leave lasting marks on history aren't remembered for their titles, but for the energy of their thoughts and the way they made others feel. It reminds me of one of my favorite sayings: **"People will forget what you said or did, but they never forget how you made them feel."** Your task is to discover your "One Thing," the unique energy you bring into the world. That is where your lasting impact lives.

Understanding energy isn't abstract philosophy; it's a practical tool for navigating daily life, medicine, and relationships. It allows us to step beyond rigid black-and-white thinking and walk comfortably in the grey. When you let go of certainty and flow with energy, you enter infinite possibility. The same force that built our galaxy also flows through you. Transformation isn't just possible; it's built into the fabric of reality.

RABBIT HOLE
Psychedelics – Ayahuasca, Psilocybin, 5-MEO-DMT

CHAPTER 8

THE POWER OF FOCUS: UNLOCKING YOUR "ONE THING"

I'll be dating myself here, but back in 1991, the movie **'City Slickers'** came out, starring Billy Crystal. There's one scene that stuck with me, even at 19 years old. Crystal's character is riding a horse with a cowboy named Curly. Curly turns to him and asks, "Do you know the secret of life?" Then he holds up one finger and says, "It's just one thing. Stick to it once you figure out what that one thing is."

That scene still moves me deeply today. As Curly said, the secret of life is discovering your "one thing" and then dedicating yourself to it, completely, every day, without hesitation. The key to becoming the best version of yourself is sharing your "one thing" with the world which creates a powerful alignment of energy within you. This energy is undistorted by emotions like fear and doubt. It's also energy that multiplies itself with power because it's in tune with your mind, body, and spirit.

Discovering and Sharpening Your "One Thing"

I challenge you to find, or rediscover, your "one thing."

What is that unique gift, passion, or purpose that motivates you even if no one notices or acknowledges it? Once you've identified it, nurture, refine, and share it without fear. This is the core of life's secret, and it's also a key to optimal health, since undistorted energy is the purest form of energy we can access. Other sources of this vital energy include love, gratitude, and joy, to name a few.

But to stay committed to your "one thing," you must first learn to observe your own thoughts. Fear from the past, or anxiety and doubt about the future, distorts your current thoughts. As Dr. Joe Dispenza would also say, "Our thoughts are for our mind, and our emotions are for our body." When you live in the present, fear and hesitation lose their grip. That's when you can show up like Santa Claus, giving away your "one thing" generously, joyfully, and without limits.

No one on their deathbed ever said, "I wish I had worked more." Instead, they regret what they didn't pursue, the love they didn't express, or the gifts they never shared. The most peaceful people I've met at the end of life are those who released rigid attachments to belief systems. They lived fully present, listening more than dictating, sharing their story without forcing it onto others.

You've probably experienced moments when someone tried to impose their beliefs upon you, or when you did the same to someone else. That's okay. The only person you're required to change is yourself.

A Lesson from My Father

My father is one of my greatest teachers on the dangers of rigid belief systems. For years, he clung tightly to his beliefs and took disagreement personally, especially from family. His defensiveness closed him off to other perspectives, creating conflict and emotional distress that eventually weighed on his health. Over time, he developed marked hearing loss, high blood pressure, a pulmonary embolism, renal carcinoma, chronic leukemia, and kidney failure requiring a transplant.

He was physically challenged, but it was equally clear that he struggled emotionally, and these difficulties often seemed to arise alongside the conflicts he faced in life. Looking back, I can see how his physical ailments were not merely biological accidents, but reflections of the toll exacted by mental and emotional rigidity. Each unresolved argument, each stubborn refusal to bend or compromise, seemed to echo inside him, creating tension that manifested in his body like a clenched fist never to open again. His conflicts with the world became conflicts within himself, blurring the line between mind and body. It was a vivid reminder that emotional patterns and belief systems don't just shape our experience, they shape our physiology, sometimes in profound ways.

Take his high blood pressure.

At first, my mom and I thought it was simply due to the standard label: "stress with work." Later, I learned it stemmed from a deeply emotional conflict where his mind signaled his body to create a new biology to respond to: elevated blood pressure.

My father was forced to retire after a surgical nurse misinterpreted his hearing issues during an operation as possible drug impairment. Poor hearing ran in his family, and as kids, my sisters and I often laughed at his misheard words. What seemed funny to us probably made him feel isolated, which I later regretted. The nurse reported her concerns, leading to a full board review. Although he was cleared of the absurd accusation (he rarely drank alcohol), the incident triggered a deeper investigation into his hearing loss and skyrocketed his malpractice insurance premiums. So on his 55th birthday, which should have been the beginning of the peak of his career, my dad was left with no choice but to retire. For him, it was a devastating loss of control over his life and career. My mom and I supported the decision, worried about his health since high blood pressure can lead to strokes or heart attacks, but at the time, I was unaware of the conflict in the background.

In Biological Decoding, hypertension reflects feelings of powerlessness and abandonment within the clan. My dad's "one thing" was being a surgeon, and in his eyes, the people within that "clan" were trying to take it away. My dad lived this conflict in real time, stripped of control over his career while the medical institution he had honored turned against him. To fight and draw attention to the conflict, the body's biological response is to raise blood flow everywhere.

And the conflicts didn't stop there.

My father, a devout Catholic, believed—though not official doctrine—that if you weren't Catholic, you went to hell. For years, I avoided confronting him, but in my mid-30s, I finally told him I no longer followed Catholicism. He didn't talk to me for two years. In his mind, I was dragging myself and my sisters, who later followed my lead, toward damnation. To him, it was a loss of sacred territory, his children's faith.

Within a year of sharing my journey of faith away from his own beliefs, his health declined further, but this time the organs involved were his kidneys.

In Biological Decoding, the kidneys represent paternal aggression, territory marking, and essential fluids. He believed that Catholicism was the "essential fluid"' for his children, and we were all three walking away from it. His anger towards me, as I mentioned earlier, became increasingly palpable over the years. My father developed kidney cancer and, a few years later, kidney failure. In 2018, he received a kidney transplant, donated by my adopted sister, that continues to support him today. He wouldn't be here without it and I don't see that as a coincidence.

Here's the point: my dad exercised regularly all his life, ate well, rarely drank, and never smoked. He had a strong marriage with my mom and several good friends. By all conventional standards, he lived a "healthy lifestyle." But underneath the surface, his emotional struggles were deep and percolating; he was the opposite of Zen.

When I shared that I had been exploring my own spiritual journey beyond Catholicism and expressing my perspective outside the boundaries he knew, it was like dropping a boulder into his pond of thought. Each interaction with me, or even with my sisters, who also lived outside of his version of strict Catholic doctrine, added more bricks to his psychological backpack. His inner rigidity combined with his external conflicts created a cascade of suffering that he projected onto all of us. Disagreements weren't just differences of opinion; they were personal affronts to his entire valued belief system.

This isn't about Catholicism itself.

It's about how tightly-held beliefs can create division within ourselves and with others. My dad had every right to his faith. But when we don't leave any room for difference, we end up building walls; walls that, in the end, imprison us and deleteriously impact our biology far more than they constrain anyone else.

Revisiting the C.A.B. Ride

Here's a simple framework to see how our own beliefs can derail us —the C.A.B. ride, revisited from my earlier example of the study on women's hormone replacement therapy:

1. **Curiosity:** gets lost when fear stops us from asking questions. Doctors, for example, once accepted a single outdated study as fact and stopped being curious about hormone replacement therapy.

2. **Awareness:** of the emotions that shape our decisions, i.e., fear of being sued.

3. **Boomerangs:** happen when fear-driven beliefs circle back, keeping patients uncertain and perpetuating outdated practices.

The Collective Consciousness and the Power of Thought

Today, information can travel at the speed of light. We can learn in nearly real-time what is happening halfway across our globe, news that in the past would have taken months. This fast flow of knowledge reflects how thoughts themselves shape reality.

As I mentioned in my first book, "Where thoughts go, energy flows." Once an idea enters human consciousness, it becomes part of our shared reality. The problem is that once it's labeled as "fact," it often goes unchallenged. Curiosity is abandoned. Cognitive dissonance takes over. But just as cell phones send signals at the speed of light, so too do our thoughts influence our biology, perhaps even faster.

Reclaiming Your "One Thing"

So how do you claim or reclaim your "one thing?" Start with three simple questions:

1. What unique gift do I offer the world?

2. What brings me my most profound joy and fulfillment?

3. What fears or rigid beliefs are holding me back from sharing it?

When you discover your "one thing," commit to it. Refine it. Share it openly. Give it away each day like Santa Claus. Doing so will align your thoughts, emotions, and energy within your body, creating a symphony of coherence for your health.

RABBIT HOLE
Human Telepathic Capacity / Remote Viewing Studies

CHAPTER 9

THE POWER OF 2%: SHIFTING CONSCIOUSNESS AND GOING VIRAL

While writing this book, I shared one of my early chapters with a patient of mine. She read it and asked me a question that stopped me cold, "How can you reach more people? I feel the masses need this so badly; it's a huge concern for our country's health." Her words hit me deep, because that's my heart, too. But then I had to check my own ego, and I was reminded of the 2% Rule.

One of the most valuable lessons I learned while writing my first book was identifying my "reading avatar." That's the imaginary reader who represents the demographics and psychographics of my ideal audience—their age, background, education, interests, beliefs, and even their cultural context. All those details matter because they shape how I choose my language, my tone, and my metaphors.

For this book, I specifically asked that very patient to review a chapter because she is my "reading avatar." She's the kind of reader I naturally connect with. Sure, I'd like to reach everyone, but here's the reality—I don't need to. Once just 2% of people adopt a new idea, the ripples begin—the "boomerang effect." After that, the idea spreads on its own. Think of it like this: I tell two people; they each tell two more, and suddenly the spark is everywhere.

If my reading avatar is young and into holistic health, I'll incorporate references to technology and long-term vision. If my avatar is older, I'll shift toward practical steps that move their health needle quickly. The point is to meet them where they are, because when the right message hits the right audience, it carries the weight that is required.

In 2012, Mark Lemley wrote, '*The Myth of the Sole Inventor*' , arguing that the idea of the <u>lone</u> genius inventor is essentially a myth. Edison didn't invent the light bulb; he improved a filament for someone else's design. Bell filed his patent for the telephone on the same day as Elisha Gray. The Wright brothers were the first to fly, but their plane barely worked and was quickly outrun by Glenn Curtiss. Lemley argued that invention is a social process, a tapestry woven from many contributors, not the triumph of a single mind.

The same principle holds true in medicine.

My "one thing" isn't about creating entirely new ideas from scratch: it's about being receptive to multiple perspectives and weaving them together. In Functional Medicine, I act as the quarterback, reading the defense and passing the ball to the right teammate for optimal physical health. In Biological Decoding, I bridge the intangible world of thoughts and emotions with the tangible reality of science in the 21st century. In essence, I assemble the work of countless brilliant minds, connecting their individual insights into a coherent, actionable whole. My "one thing" is being a kind of puzzle player for medicine.

Now, let's talk numbers. My reading avatar represents about 14% of the U.S. population, roughly 47 million people. To reach the tipping point of 2%, this book would need to connect with around 9 million U.S. readers. Will I accomplish that alone? Probably not. But that's the point—I'm not alone. Just as Dr. Jeff Bland wasn't alone with Functional Medicine, I stand on the shoulders of those who came before me and alongside others now, such as my mentor Isabelle Benarous, who continues the work of Dr. Hamer and Dr. Sabbah.

Every revolutionary idea follows a similar path: first, it's dismissed as "quackery," then tolerated as "a possibility," and eventually integrated into mainstream beliefs. I've experienced this myself.

That is why I talk about taking a **C.A.B. Ride** of your own thoughts and beliefs often:

1. **C**uriosity: Become curious about the thought(s) behind your emotion.

2. **A**wareness: of the precise emotion, where you feel it, and

how it feels.

3. **B**oomerang: What kind of energy are you sending out?

Without curiosity and awareness, we can hinder innovative thought and ideas with our own boomerangs of dismissiveness, which are the opposite of growth. In the world of Biological Decoding, if we fail to take a **C.A.B Ride**, we can unknowingly create gaps of divisive thinking attached to emotions, leading to our own internal "conflicts." This is not to suggest that we are supposed to agree with or even lean into every idea, but instead, it's about leaving room for the concept of all possibilities, creating an ocean within our psyche rather than a pond that can be disturbed and triggered by even the smallest dropped pebbles.

During my final year of Family Medicine residency, a physician colleague and I served as co-chief residents. She and I were close friends. After graduation, our career paths diverged significantly. She worked only outpatient two days a week while raising children, whereas I joined a progressive group of five other physicians who served as the town's primary providers for everything. We kept in touch over the years, but our experiences as physicians could not have been more different, and the distance between how we each thought about medicine became increasingly evident whenever we reconnected.

She was a strong advocate for Family Medicine, and when I later mentioned exploring Functional Medicine, her tone and connection with me grew noticeably more distant. When I wrote my first book, I asked her to read it, hoping to hear her thoughts. To my disappointment, she said she hadn't read it because she felt she already knew enough about Functional Medicine from others and did not believe in it.

When I pressed further, she admitted she didn't want to elaborate because she assumed I was only seeking her validation. That was far from the truth. I wanted to share my work with her because I believed we were friends first. Yet, the way she talked about medicine revealed how, even as a doctor, she had become almost an NPC—a thinker on autopilot. When she spoke, she sounded like someone stuck in a medical mindset that had barely evolved since our initial training, even after twenty years. When physicians do that, it also limits the growth of our patients' well-being and development.

What I realized is that she was always avoiding discussing anything new I had to share. That avoidance, and the distance I felt from her, came from a fear of subjects she knew little about, a fear of being exposed as not knowing enough, and a fear of being seen as less than the label we carry. Many doctors live under that label, believing they must know everything, which prevents them from exploring outside ideas. I understand this because I felt it myself; for the first five years after becoming a physician, I resisted being called "doctor" because I feared everyone would expect me to have all the answers. Today, I push back a little against being called a doctor since labels, whether we claim them or others assign them, can quietly restrict growth.

In her case, she viewed Family and Functional Medicine not as complementary but as opposite paths. Her strong loyalty to Family Medicine was an unwavering belief; yet, that loyalty created a barrier, preventing her from seeing how the two could coexist and benefit each other. With her ego in the driver's seat, it sent her emotions of fear, distrust, and disloyalty. Sadly, she severed our friendship.

Rigid friends, rigid colleagues, rigid family members, rigid thinkers —they'll keep you boxed in. Expanding into the grey will create friction, because it forces others to confront their own rigidity. But that's the price of evolving.

Now, let me lighten it up with a real-life example of going viral.

During a recent trip to Mexico, my teenage daughter filmed a TikTok. She wore a hand-painted fedora she had made with her mom, with the brim decorated in colorful brushstrokes and small designs, making it unique. With a trending song playing in the background, she strolled through the resort, pointing at palm trees, the pool, the beach, and the staff, all synchronized with the beat. The staff laughed and joined in, one even leaping into frame with a wave, while my wife filmed the scene, walking backward to avoid tripping over lounge chairs. The atmosphere was relaxed and fun, just pure, joyful energy packed into 15 seconds.

She had about 1,000 followers at the time. Day one: the video hit 1 million views. Day two: 8 million. Suddenly, she had 10,000 followers, comments from strangers all over the world, and brands sliding into her DMs. As her dad, my first thought was, "WTF?!" My second thought was: *"**This is the 2% effect in action.**"*

Her video crossed the threshold and the growth was exponential. Two percent doubled to 4%, then 8%, then 16%. By 10 million views, she had touched around 30% of her demographic worldwide. That's the power of resonance.

But here's the twist: within three days, her "fame" faded. The algorithm moved on. Yet unlike TikTok trends, when an idea goes viral in human consciousness, it lingers. Even if it fades from the spotlight, it remains stored and accessible to anyone who searches for it. Just as nothing truly disappears online, perhaps nothing ever truly vanishes from human thought either. Maybe that's why there are "no new thoughts," only rediscoveries of old ones.

So, whether it's through a book, a podcast, a medical practice, or a TikTok, every thought we share becomes part of the collective. Each boomerang influences the future in ways we might never fully realize.

RABBIT HOLE
The Akashic Records

CHAPTER 10

THE VIRAL NATURE OF THOUGHT: HOW SHIFTS IN CONSCIOUSNESS SHAPE OUR WORLD

When collective human consciousness shifts, the world changes, often quickly. Yet, in the moment, it can feel subtle... until you look around and wonder, **"How did we get here?"**

Take Kim Kardashian.

Her influence reshaped modern beauty standards. The focus shifted from breasts to the booty. Weight rooms once filled with men now host women deadlifting and squatting with barbells. Plastic surgeons pivoted from breast implants to Brazilian butt lifts. Fashion followed suit, spotlighting curves over thinness.

This "new" ideal wasn't new to every culture, but Kim brought it to global consciousness, and that's the key. She didn't invent the trend; **she made it mainstream**. A shift in collective thought made it real.

That's how ideas shape reality.

I remember the first time I saw a website URL on a billboard in the 1990s and told my dad, "This www-dot thing is going to be big." Today, the internet shapes our lives. Landlines and phone booths are now outdated. Electric vehicle charging stations briefly appeared in the early '90s and then disappeared, only to come back when Tesla revolutionized the industry. Before 1953, a sub-4-minute mile seemed impossible, then one man did it, and now thousands have. Every big change starts with a thought—a whisper of possibility. Once that idea reaches critical mass, once belief shifts, it no longer seems unlikely. **It becomes the new normal.**

Paradigm shifts don't just change the world - they change us

When I first discovered Functional Medicine, it seemed to sharply conflict with everything I knew from Western medicine. Traditional training taught me to manage symptoms, while Functional Medicine encouraged me to identify root causes. At first, I felt like I was betraying my profession. I was excited by the possibilities but also overwhelmed with regret. I had spent years mastering a system I now saw as incomplete for chronic care. The internal conflict was genuinely difficult. Eventually, I stopped viewing them as opposing ideologies and realized that these are thought patterns related to different parts of the same book. Both are valuable and necessary. Together, they provide a more complete understanding of health and healing.

But not everyone gets to that point.

Many physicians avoid facing this kind of shift. It threatens their identity, training, and livelihood. It demands emotional effort they don't have the time or bandwidth for. They might explore new paradigms, such as Functional Medicine, Energy Medicine, or Biological Decoding, but when emotional tension rises, they tend to withdraw. And I don't blame them. I've been through it.

But this resistance comes with a price: we end up focusing on treating disease rather than healing people.

This isn't a criticism; it's a call for compassion. The fear of being wrong, starting over, and stepping into unfamiliar territory extends far beyond physicians. It's real life. At my lowest point, I even considered leaving medicine because I didn't think I could practice the principles of Functional Medicine within the constraints of conventional medical design. But that's when I realized they were not in opposition but complemented each other. I chose instead to create something new—a system that honored both worlds. That integration became my peace and my patients' greatest benefit.

Thought quality going viral

That's why being an "influencer" is so seductive, especially to younger generations. They see, almost addictively, how fast ideas can spread. One video. One quote. One post, and suddenly, the world sees things differently.

But there's a catch.

Just like a virus, every thought carries consequences. Every idea you "share" ripples outward and returns. The **C.A.B. ride** helps keep this in check:

1. **C**uriosity: about the thought's <u>intention</u>

2. **A**wareness: of the emotion it stirs

3. **B**oomerang: the ripple effect it has on others and back to you

If you spread fear, division, or outrage into the collective, it *WILL* come back amplified. In today's world, we recognize that fear is a powerful sales tool. **An odd aspect of human nature is that we are motivated by joy and desire, but we are often encouraged through fear and pain.**

During the COVID-19 pandemic, I warned my patients about this. The media's relentless fear campaigns created a tangible, global stress response. Guess what suppresses the immune system? Chronic stress.

Every one of my patients eventually contracted COVID. Most

experienced it more than once. But those who stayed grounded and resisted fear recovered faster and more completely. Those who immersed themselves in anxiety and media panic stayed longer in illness. Some developed long COVID. The difference was striking and unfortunately predictable.

It echoes a core truth I wrote about in my first book: **"Where thoughts go, energy flows."**

Biological Decoding emphasizes the mind-body connection more sharply, **explaining that unresolved emotional conflicts**, especially those rooted in internal contradictions, **can manifest physically in a specific organ,** following a kind of emotional map in the brain.

The part of the brain that activates depends on the emotion and how your subconscious symbolically interprets it. For example, if something feels too overwhelming to "digest," your stomach might be affected since digestion is a biological process. You may have even experienced irritable bowel syndrome yourself and can easily recognize when you experience it during times of stress, in particular. The brain acts as a map of the body, providing an understanding of the mind-body connection between a specific conflict and an organ, but it is the energy of a deeply powerful emotion that influences gene expression within that organ.

Gene expression is the process by which our genes produce

proteins that tell our cells what to do. For example, if the body wants to boost digestion, it will increase both the size and activity of the cells that produce stomach acid. While this helps digestion biologically, it can also lead to excess acid, causing heartburn or reflux.

In conventional Western medicine, the usual approach is to prescribe acid-reducing medications. However, in Functional Medicine, we look deeper, we search for the **S.T.A.M.P**. triggers that make the stomach more vulnerable to overproduction, such as food sensitivities or alcohol. In Biological Decoding, the focus shifts yet again. Here, we explore the underlying "conflict" that precedes everything, triggering the gene to initially over-express or even under-express from the very beginning.

Thoughts trigger emotions, and emotions shape biology. Yes, that's a giant leap from conventional medicine. And no, I don't expect you to fully believe it. But I invite you to stay curious. Notice how this may already be playing out in your life and the lives of those you love. The pandemic, after all, was more than just a health crisis. It was a consciousness crisis.

Conflicting thoughts flooded the collective mind. Controversies over treatments like hydroxychloroquine and ivermectin weren't just medical; they were political, personal, and highly divisive. States like California and Florida became opposite ends of a consciousness spectrum. Even families were split over beliefs. Scientists had to innovate in real-time, balancing new data from established norms while facing unprecedented pressure.

As a physician, this demanded more flexibility than I'd ever needed. I had to re-learn how to listen, who to trust, and how to protect my own peace while navigating conflicting truths. And here's what I learned: **Viral thoughts, accurate or not, don't just shape society; they can also shape biology at an organ level.**

So, I leave you with this: What kind of thought waves are you sending out? Are you influencing your work with love, curiosity, and connection? Or are you driven by fear, division, and programmed NPC scripts? Because the thoughts we nurture today will shape the world we inherit tomorrow.

RABBIT HOLE
Brain Spotting / EMDR

CHAPTER 11

THE ANATOMY OF THOUGHT: HOW EMOTIONS SHAPE BIOLOGY

By now, you should have a deeper understanding of how disease, when reverse-engineered, often reveals its origins in the power of a belief—a thought connected to a deeply rooted emotion. But how do we transform the quantum energy of a thought, tied to a specific emotion, into biology?

Let's start with a relatable example.

Ask someone where they were during 9/11 or when the COVID-19 shutdown was announced. Watch their eyes closely. Most people will glance up and to the left as they retrieve memories from the "file cabinets" of their brains. Now, ask a question you think they might not answer honestly, and watch their eyes, often darting to the upper right, a common sign of creative thinking. But don't jump to conclusions; this eye movement doesn't always mean lying, it could simply indicate boredom or dismissiveness. For fun, ask a younger person, too young to remember 9/11, the same question and observe their eye movements. These subtle changes reveal a fascinating truth: thoughts have distinct "file cabinets" in our brains, often tagged with emotions. (Quick tip: if someone is left-handed, these directions can be reversed.)

This book plants a critical seed: **your beliefs create your biology.**

I'm not going to delve into each complex science here, such as neuroimmunology, neuroendocrinology, epigenetics, gene expression, and post-transcriptional gene editing, which are just a few areas already explored in detail. Instead, I'm here to help connect all these puzzle pieces by applying the framework of Biological Decoding to understand how thoughts and emotions influence biology by engaging the "C" in your **C.A.B. ride.** Curiosity will guide you, helping you see how your thoughts affect your health and physiology. And if this sparks even 2% of human consciousness to ask more profound questions about Biological Decoding...well, I did my part.

The Science of Thought Meets Biology

Thoughts influence biology through three primary pathways:

1. Neuro-chemical pathways

2. Neuro-electrical pathways

3. Neuro-immune-endocrine pathways

At its core, **neuro-chemical** studies focus on how the brain transforms emotional thought energy (a belief) into biological processes through chemical messengers like serotonin. For example, my mom's Prozac increased serotonin to influence her emotions. But here's the catch: changing chemistry alone doesn't release the lingering quantum energy linked to the emotion or how it is stored in our super subconscious fabric. That unresolved energy is like a brick in your psychological backpack; it becomes a weight that affects your biology until it's released. If fixing emotions were as simple as tweaking one neurotransmitter, we would have solved mental illness long ago.

Neuro-electrical studies examine how thoughts and emotions influence the body's electrical system, which is part of our nervous system. You may be familiar with the main pathways: the parasympathetic system, responsible for rest, relaxation, and healing, and the sympathetic system, involved in the fight-or-flight response. Techniques such as deep breathing, sound bowl therapy, cold immersion, or visualization affect the vagus nerve, the long wandering nerve connecting the brain to the organs, shifting these pathways and regulating your body's "circuit board."

Neuro-immune-endocrine studies explore how thoughts influence hormonal release and coordinate our defenses, collectively referred to as our immune system. Take cortisol, the stress hormone, as an example. In moderation, cortisol builds resilience. But if the stress "button" is stuck on, it wreaks havoc, weakening immunity, disrupting sleep, and paving the way for chronic disease.

A story from my early training highlights this. One of my attending physicians enjoyed quizzing us on the 16 major side effects of long-term prednisone, a synthetic cortisol. We listed them: memory impairment/brain fog, mood swings, anxiety, depression, sleep issues, headaches, fragile skin, blurred vision, thrush, GI problems, suppressed immunity, high blood sugar, weight gain, increased blood pressure, fatigue, osteoporosis, and muscle loss.

Sound familiar?

Chronic stress can produce the same effects. Prednisone can be lifesaving in the short term but may cause serious damage over time. Similarly, unresolved emotional "bricks" continue to activate cortisol without awareness. I've seen many patients with chronic fatigue, brain fog, anxiety, or weight gain. Ignoring their unresolved emotional conflicts often sabotages their complete healing. The World Health Organization reports that 90% of office visits today are attributed to "stress."

Why me? Why did I get this disease?

Dr. Bruce Lipton conducted groundbreaking research on stem cells at Stanford University School of Medicine, showing that the environment around a cell, not just its genes, can influence gene activity. When genetic determinism was the dominant scientific belief, his findings challenged traditional ideas and helped establish the field of epigenetics. Although Lipton eventually left academia, he dedicated himself to sharing these insights with a wider audience through books and lectures, making complex cellular biology understandable and impactful, especially in his influential work, *The Biology of Belief*.

Lipton's research shows how a series of chemical, electrical, and hormonal signals ultimately come together at the cellular level. In *The Biology of Belief*, he describes the cell membrane as acting like a computer chip, collecting signals through receptors and deciding how the cell responds based on the proteins it creates. These proteins, in turn, give instructions that shape our biology. Lipton, who also wrote my medical school's *Cell Biology* textbook, was one of the first to prove the principles of epigenetics, revealing decades before it became widely accepted how environment, perception, and energy influence gene expression and overall health.

Epigenetics explores how signals "above" the genes control gene expression. The Human Genome Project (HGP) revealed that humans have about 20,000 genes; however, before its completion, it was known that our bodies produce around 100,000 proteins. A gene is not a one-size-fits-all protein maker. Yes, genes create proteins. A protein acts as a dynamic set of various instruction manuals for possibilities influenced by epigenetic signals from thoughts, emotions, and biological environment signals that gather on the cell membrane, much like a marinade.

When the Human Genome Project concluded in 2003, scientists realized humans have fewer genes than a rat. This discrepancy sparked deeper exploration into how a single gene can create hundreds (likely thousands) of variations via post-transcriptional RNA splicing.

Returning to the copy machine analogy from Chapter 6, if we asked for 100 copies of a document, do you think they would all look the same? The copy machine itself would have a margin of error caused by dirty glass (also known as aging via telomere shortening), which can create copying artifacts, as well as by the amount of toner available for each copy. Yet, the copy machine is also capable of producing nearly identical copies when it is properly maintained and serviced.

The same is true for the protein a gene decides to produce. The "copy" from the gene can also differ from the original, resulting in millions of protein variants through mechanisms like alternative splicing and SNPs (single-nucleotide polymorphisms). These concepts go beyond the scope of this book, but I encourage you to explore them further.

By 2019, it was estimated that humans could produce up to 4.7 million proteoforms, influenced by genetic and cellular signaling. Today, discoveries of new proteins and their isoforms are cataloged in the Human Proteome Project, a universal database maintained by the Human Proteome Organization (HUPO). However, it's essential to acknowledge that the working hypothesis I favor is that the protein ultimately produced is shaped by the signals triggered by our thoughts and emotions. It's not just my belief in this hypothesis, but also what I observe clinically in my patients along with many other physicians worldwide, who report similar findings. This reinforces Biological Decoding as a viable and reliable framework for understanding this process and working through the questions a person asks when they are first diagnosed with a disease: Why me? What caused this to happen to me in the first place?

Zooming Out

Our conscious thoughts, along with their attached subconscious emotions and memories, are drawn from the "file cabinets" of memory and create a ripple effect that shapes our biology. Here's the basic sequence:

1. Thoughts and their attached emotions, aka our beliefs, are

energy, rippling outward like a stone dropped in a pond.

2. This energy triggers a "marinade" of neuro-chemical, neuro-electrical, and neuro-immune-endocrine signals.

3. The signal marinade converges at the cellular membrane, influencing which protein will be produced.

4. Gene expression selects from multiple protein instruction options, ultimately shaping biology to mirror the original thought and its deep-seated emotions metaphorically in biological terms, influenced heavily by our subconscious programming.

Unresolved emotional conflicts can disrupt balance, sending ripples through physiology. The anatomy of thought becomes the biology of thought, profoundly influencing health. Here's the takeaway: by resolving conflicts and aligning your thoughts with your authentic mind, body, and spirit, you can impact emotional well-being and physical health at every level.

RABBIT HOLE
Eckhart Tolle – Mindfulness Training

CHAPTER 12

WHY ME? WHY DID I GET THIS DISEASE? MEET KAREN

Now that the foundation is in place, the real work and the real intrigue begin as we explore stories from actual patients.

Thoughts and emotions are energy. Both transform into biological signals, creating a "marinade" that bathes our cell membranes and influences which proteins are expressed from our genes. This marinade subtly alters the instructions, aligning our beliefs with our biology.

To dismiss thoughts as irrelevant is a mistake. Evaluating the quality of our thoughts is not just important; it's essential, given how deeply they shape our biology. To show how subtle yet profound this influence can be, let me share the story of a patient. I'll call her Karen. (Yes, I know, classic meme name. But stay with me.)

Karen was 47 when she was diagnosed with right-sided breast cancer. The news stunned her, her family, and everyone who knew her. Outwardly, she looked like the picture of health. She wasn't just fit, she was ripped. She ate clean, organic, whole foods and avoided processed ingredients. She exercised regularly, had strong relationships, especially with her husband and children, and described herself as having a consistently positive outlook.

Fortunately, her cancer was caught early and required only minimal surgery. She was prescribed medication to reduce recurrence risk over the next decade. That's when she came to see me.

Karen's mission was clear; she wanted to go deeper. Beyond what was obviously in her control, she wanted to uncover: **Why me?** Why had she developed cancer in the first place, and how could she prevent it from returning? Like many patients, she assumed the root cause would be physical, something in her diet, her environment, or her lab results. Together, we left no stone unturned.

The Investigation Starts

We began systematically, starting in Karen's kitchen and focusing on her hormone balance. Using the **S.T.A.M.P.** framework, **S**tressors, **T**oxins, **A**llergens, **M**icrobes, and **P**oor diet, we explored every possible angle. These are the exact steps I outline in my first book, *Functional Medicine: The New Standard*.

We examined broad and specific biomarkers, connecting each result with potential triggers. But nothing stood out.

Karen insisted she wasn't stressed, and her physical health looked impeccable. At that point, it was time to revisit her "book of disease", the chapters that reveal the origins of her illness as reflected in her beliefs. I asked her about her thoughts and any emotionally charged events in the 6 to 12 months before her diagnosis, the critical window when unresolved conflicts often simmer before becoming physical illness, shaping what has been described as "new biology." That's when the veil began to lift.

At first, Karen hesitated. But eventually, she opened up about something she had never shared, not with me, not with her husband, and not even with her closest friends. About nine months before her diagnosis, her teenage child came out to her as gay. It was an emotional, private conversation. Her child begged her not to tell their father, fearing his reaction.

Karen suddenly found herself in a painful emotional conflict.

She wanted to honor her child's trust, but she also felt guilty for hiding this from her husband, with whom she had a close bond. She hadn't considered this a "stressor" at the time, nor had she connected it to her cancer. But as she reflected, the weight of her internal struggle became undeniable. She was torn between protecting her child's secret and remaining loyal to her husband through honesty. That silent tug of war pressed on her heart and mind in the months leading up to her diagnosis.

The Emotional Weight

Karen was determined to do everything possible to understand and prevent her cancer from returning. That meant facing her conflicting beliefs head-on, protecting her child's confidence versus staying transparent with her husband. She admitted the secrecy still felt like carrying bricks in her emotional backpack. Her story revealed how guilt and shame had been quietly simmering beneath the surface, influencing her biology without her even realizing it.

As Karen shared this with me, I could see a physical shift in her body and face. Once she connected the dots between her emotional conflict and her cancer, she described the experience as both humbling and empowering. It was as if those heavy bricks had finally been lifted.

This realization changed everything.

Karen later had an open conversation with her child, sharing the emotional chains of guilt and shame that had silently poisoned her and contributed to her illness. It wasn't about blaming her child; it was about releasing her own burden. Thankfully, more than 18 months had passed, and her child was now ready to share their truth with their father. That moment liberated Karen completely.

Since then, she has not only avoided recurrence but, more importantly, has gained deep confidence that it will not return, rooted in her profound understanding of her own intuition.

The Science Behind Karen's Story

I can already hear critics asking, **"How do you know her cancer won't come back?" "How do you know this was the cause of her cancer?"** The answer is straightforward but somewhat incomplete. Quantum physics has demonstrated that we are connected by a vast, all-encompassing energetic field that permeates everything. And everything within this great field also has its own fields. Those fields influence other fields. Since we know that everything is made of energy and that beliefs carry energy, it's the most convincing science explaining how biology doesn't follow simple cause-and-effect rules but is influenced through a mixture of epigenetic signals, offering a range of possibilities and probabilities of gene expression. It also aligns more closely with the Placebo Effect and the findings from the Blue Zones than any physical explanation in Conventional or Functional Medicine.

Modern medicine is good at treating symptoms, identifying mutations, and managing disease. However, it often falls short of clearly explaining the upstream triggers that influence gene expression from the start. Epigenetics has shown that our environment, lifestyle, and even emotional states can affect which genes are turned on. Chronic stress, unresolved trauma, or persistent negative thoughts are forms of energetic and chemical signals that can change cellular function, immune responses, and hormone regulation over time.

Biological Decoding **offers a thought framework** for understanding these subtle influences by linking subconscious programming and emotional patterns to the biological pathways that can contribute to disease. It examines not just the "what" of illness but also the "why" behind each patient's physiological responses. Through this thought model, we gain a deeper, more holistic understanding of health and potential interventions.

Karen's story shows, with the highest clarity so far, how disease can develop when the body's delicate signaling system gets disrupted, like dropping a boulder into a pond of consciousness. This boulder of emotion creates the "marinade" of biological signals, which end at the cell membrane and eventually affect the genes. The proteins made from those genes respond to the initial boulder, trying to create biology that symbolically matches.

In Karen's story, her breast symbolizes femininity as an organ, representing motherhood and wifehood, which is where her "conflict" lives. The right side is a symbolic reflection of others besides her mother, who would be linked to the left side. This was first observed by Dr. Hamer, who attempted to reverse-engineer the stories behind hundreds of breast cancer cases. Since then, many followers have expanded on his original paradigm of a quantum leap of thought. I will be the first to admit we still have a long way to go, but current advances in genetics and epigenetics provide remarkable evidence.

Genes themselves are static; they serve as the blueprint. However, **epigenetics**, which involves signals "above" the genes and what we now understand through post-transcriptional editing, determines which proteins those genes produce. When these signals are mixed with signals of negative emotions rather than restorative thoughts, the body is forced to adapt and construct a new biology—one that better reflects this "new" layer of signals.

This creates a biology that aligns with the symbolism within our subconscious programs, as described by Dr. Sabbah's work on creating cancer, as seen in Karen. Her body was trying to match her thoughts with her biology by producing a larger version of her identity as a mom and wife, specifically, by creating an overgrowth of cells in her breast called cancer.

In Karen's case, her right breast became the focus. Her guilt and shame were linked to specific emotional thoughts stored in a particular part of her brain. The brain, acting as a roadmap to the body, directed these negative signals to her breast tissue metaphorically. This is an example of Biological Decoding, where emotions and thoughts (also known as beliefs) are connected to specific organs, creating new biology within those organs that we refer to as disease.

When Karen released her emotional conflict, the signals to her breast shifted, returning to a biology more consistent with typical breast biology. This release, which was palpable when I worked with Karen, severed the invisible cord of her thoughts that created her cancer.

Biological Decoding is simply a thought template, not necessarily the final answer to the origins of disease. However, it provides a framework that guides all relevant modern sciences more logically. For those who incorporate the **C.A.B. rides** with their intuitive senses and align them with current sciences, it elevates the question everyone asks, **"Why me? Why did I get this disease?"**, from pseudoscience to at least the realm of "possibility."

I invite you to stay with me. I warned you that this book would stretch your comfort levels and belief systems.

The idea that thoughts create our biology is not new. Biological Decoding has just gift-wrapped it more intentionally and thoughtfully. It aligns perfectly with the work of physicians who have dedicated their careers to studying the "miracles" of medicine, the common thread being how a patient transformed their mindset, which reversed their disease. We see this in the work of heart-brain coherence studies with people like Dr. Joe Dispenza or the work of the Heart-Math Institute.

We also observe this in researchers who are deeply interested in the causal factors affecting the people living in the Blue Zones. These are regions on Earth that have the highest percentage of people who live to be over 100 years old. A common feature across these areas is that residents report a shared purpose and a strong sense of community, which enhances their emotional and mental well-being.

Finally, as I mentioned earlier, every major high-quality study is compared to a placebo. Interestingly, the placebo effect, which occurs when one believes they are receiving something while receiving nothing, results in healing in nearly every study conducted.

The Power of Connecting our Thoughts to our Emotions

The most compelling evidence of this connection isn't just the science; it was the visible, palpable shift in Karen's face, eyes, and body language when she made the connection. The release of carrying her child's belief was visceral.

We need to move beyond the black-and-white thinking that dominates modern medicine. While evidence-based research is essential, it often overlooks the vital role of emotions, thoughts, and belief systems— factors usually grouped into the "placebo effect" that remains undiscussed or simplified as "stress," or worse, dismissed by a lazy NPC as "crazy."

Many fail to see that placebo patients improve because they engage their quantum thoughts and emotions. This isn't a coincidence; it's biology in action. Karen's story is a testament to the power of addressing the emotional roots of disease. We can reclaim control over our health by connecting to our origin story.

RABBIT HOLE
IV Ketamine Therapy – Treatment of PTSD and
Recalcitrant Depression

CHAPTER 13

DECODING KAREN: SYNTHESIZING HER C.A.B. RIDE TO DISEASE

Let's break down the story of Karen. On the surface, she seemed to embody health by societal standards, both physically and mentally, for the most part. But there was still an unresolved conflict; even in her mindfulness, she downplayed something much more significant than herself, yet her body didn't forget.

In Karen's situation, she failed to take the **C.A.B. ride** with all her thoughts. Instead, she built an emotional brick of unresolved conflict linked to shame and guilt, downplaying its importance. We all do this; I've done this, too. The key is learning how to release these deep-rooted emotions before they become unconscious, epigenetic signals that change our body's "marinade" of signals, leading to a biology that isn't beneficial.

This process requires mastering the **C.A.B. ride,** a mental framework to process thoughts tied to strong emotions. Let me recap the steps once again:

1. **C**uriosity: Get curious about the thought(s) behind your emotion

2. **A**wareness: of your precise emotion, where you feel it in your body, and what it feels like

3. **B**oomerang: understand the energy you put out in response that will hit others and you in the head 3-fold

Hindsight is always 20/20, but let's re-imagine how Karen could have applied the **C.A.B. ride** process that might have derailed her biology toward her breast cancer.

When her child confided that they were gay and asked her not to share this with their dad, it created an enormous conflict between protecting her child's confidentiality and sharing with her husband, whom she never liked to keep secrets, especially regarding their child. If she had paused to get **C**urious about her original emotion, she would have asked herself: "What is the thought behind my emotion?"

Next, she could have directed her **A**wareness inward, asking herself: "What is the most precise emotion I am feeling? Where do I feel it in my body? What does it feel like?" When she and I took these steps in retrospect together, she felt guilt and shame centered in her heart, like a heavy ache.

This realization led to a crucial insight: her fear, shame, and guilt were not her own. They stemmed from her child's own fear of their dad's reaction, which then caused shame and guilt when hearing this news. As a result, she kept this secret from her husband as a burden, aiming to protect all three of them.

She "held it close to her chest to protect her child," literally and figuratively. This is where the emotional "brick" settled in her backpack for her to carry for her child. This was the emotional "conflict" that challenged the alignment in her otherwise healthy body.

Finally, the **B**oomerang of emotion hit her every single day. She felt guilt whenever she looked at her child and her husband. It was an endless loop of shame and guilt that weighed on her physically, emotionally, and energetically.

Had Karen taken this **C.A.B. ride** earlier, it wouldn't have erased all her emotions, but it would have brought clarity. She would have realized that many of the feelings she was experiencing weren't truly hers, but belonged to her child, layered with the child's fear of how their father might react.

That awareness alone could have eased her emotional burden and reduced the physiological stress she was experiencing. With that understanding, she might have started a conversation with her child sooner, helping them feel safe enough to talk with their father and, in turn, changing the emotional "marinade" within her body that had been poisoning her for months.

Once I helped Karen view her story as an observer of herself, you could see the guillotine fall, severing the toxic ties of her thoughts and emotions to her breast.

C.A.B. Rides and Daily Life

This process isn't just about preventing disease; it's about healthier relationships. When we are in healthy relationships with those around us, these relationships boomerang far beyond our conceptualized world. But it requires us to take a **C.A.B. ride** with every thought that evokes a powerful emotion. It does not have to be at the level Karen experienced.

Let me share a recent example from my own life.

One night, our teenage daughter asked me to drive her to her weekly church service. Oddly enough, it had just snowed in Houston—a rare six inches! I told her I thought it was best to avoid the roads at night since they could get icy, and honestly, I wasn't feeling up to the late-night drive to pick her up either. Later, she texted me to say she found a friend's dad to carpool with, and I agreed since the roads looked fine after all. So off to church she went.

Fast forward to 8:30 p.m. I'm chilling on the couch when my wife comes rushing downstairs with keys in hand, already one foot out the door. Surprised, I ask her what she's doing. She tells me, obviously annoyed, that she needed to pick up our daughter.

Suddenly, I felt a surge of anger. I texted our daughter irritably and asked firmly, "What happened to your carpool?" She casually texts me back, "Oh, he canceled, so I asked mom to pick me up. It's not a big deal, Dad."

Cue the fury rising inside me. My gut reaction was to text her back and tell her how frustrated I was. But this time, I decided to sit with it until she arrived home and take my own **C.A.B. ride**.

I got curious: What is the thought behind my anger? Through curiosity, I separated myself from the situation. I transferred my thoughts from my reptilian brain to my frontal cortex, creating a space bubble for more rational, higher-level thinking.

Then, I turned my awareness inward.

What exactly is the emotion I am feeling? I was angry, but I have realized that anger, fear, or even depression is always something more profound. I realized I was feeling duped, like she had manipulated the situation, by going behind my back to her mom. I also felt hurt by her lack of empathy, as she had made her mom drive late at night after her mom had specifically asked to sit this one out. I noticed the physical sensation of my emotions, an empty, churning feeling in my gut. In my mind, the conclusion was that she lied, manipulated, and didn't care how this affected her mom or me.

In the past, my boomerang would have been an angry outburst, marked by a raised voice, choice words, and a sharp tone. But this time, I created space for myself to process. Once clear, I walked into the room where my daughter sat and calmly shared my thoughts and emotions. I expressed my specific feelings, the reasons behind them, without anger or blame.

To my surprise (but not really) she responded with maturity and empathy. She said she understood and would be more thoughtful next time. That was it. The boomerang I sent out came back as respect.

Why the C.A.B. Rides Matter

I encourage you to take as many intentional **C.A.B. rides** as possible. Whether it's to prevent disease or foster healthier relationships, the outcome remains the same: clarity, emotional release, better relationships, and optimal biology. Sometimes, the stakes are as high as the difference between health and illness. Other times, the rewards are even more significant: a deeper, more genuine connection with the people you love. By setting a clear intention to take the necessary C.A.B. rides, you can improve the quality of your life, making it more rewarding and fulfilling.

RABBIT HOLE

Dr. Joe Dispenza and others – *Heal*, documentary available on Netflix

CHAPTER 14

CHANGING ENERGY THROUGH LOVE: THE HIGHEST FORM OF EMOTIONAL ENERGY

Part of our human "code" involves giving and receiving love. Dr. Gary Chapman's book, *The Five Love Languages* describes five primary ways we express love:

    1. Words of Affirmation

    2. Physical Touch

    3. Quality Time

    4. Acts of Service

    5. Receiving Gifts

We all appreciate each aspect, but one or two usually dominate. For me, it's Words of Affirmation and Physical Touch. I can trace this back to my mom, who constantly hugged me and told me she loved me; it became one of the primary languages by which I feel most seen and validated.

My dad's love languages are Acts of Service and Quality Time.

While those are valuable, they do not resonate as deeply with me. I longed to hear affirming words or feel the connection of a spontaneous hug from my dad, but those were few and far between, leaving me feeling unseen by my dad in the ways that mattered to me.

We often express love in our preferred language, assuming others will receive it the same way. But to truly connect, we need to learn their language. It's like hacking into their energy grid. People give you what they wish to receive. If the person you care about most in the world showers you with gifts, then shower them with gifts. It's the boomerang they are asking for from you.

It may not always feel natural since it's not your love language, but with some practice, you can start to see what sticks and how a little intention goes a long way to creating an environment with more love and intention.

Reflect for a moment to answer the following:

- How do your loved ones show you love?

- Are you expressing love in their language or yours?

This slight but intentional shift can create an enormous ripple effect in your relationships.

Consciousness Beyond the Collective – Break the Labels

Understanding love languages goes far beyond romantic relationships; it's about reshaping the energy you bring into the world. Take something as simple as a hug. I've always greeted people with hugs, whether men or women. But in the 1980s, hugging another man was taboo. I can still feel the awkward tension from those moments, the hesitation as if we were breaking some unspoken rule. Yet, I kept hugging, refusing to let those invisible boundaries define me.

By the time I reached my 20s, the resistance seemed to fade. Hugging had become more acceptable, even expected. Did my persistence play a small part in shifting this social "code?" In my little corner of the world, I like to think so.

Think about it: what small decisions have you made that changed the energy in your environment? Maybe you've chosen to offer genuine gratitude in a workplace where appreciation is rare or to greet neighbors with a smile when others barely make eye contact. Even subtle actions like these can ripple outward, transforming a room, a team, or a community.

In my work as a physician, I've learned to tailor my energy to those around me. I lean on tools like personality frameworks, such as the Myers-Briggs test. If someone is more logic-driven, I speak in structures and facts. If they're more emotion-driven, I tap into feelings and empathy. I interact with people as if writing to their reading avatar. However, while these tools can guide us, we must also exercise caution. Labels are double-edged swords, whether assigned by society, family, or even by yourself.

I'll use myself as an example. I'm a white male; this is my social and genetic identity, not an achievement. I'm a physician–a profession, not my identity. I'm a husband, a role I've chosen. Each label carries meaning, shaped by the collective views of our time. In a different era, I might have had five wives. Today, that choice would break the social code, leading to a cascade of consequences and an even more complex social structure.

But here's the danger: if we can only identify and interact with others through our labels, we risk building a life that looks successful on the surface but feels hollow inside. This misalignment, the disconnect between our life and the life our soul craves, can quietly erode our energy and sense of purpose, and unconsciously create an unfavorable biology.

When I started my Family Medicine residency in conservative Omaha, Nebraska in 2000, I suddenly faced the unspoken expectation to wear a tie while working in the hospital. My wife jokes that I look and act stiff when I wear anything formal, especially a tie. She says I am visibly uncomfortable. That's true. The idea of wearing a tie for a 36-hour shift over the next three years felt like a personal hell, like a colorful, respectable noose around my neck.

Within a few months of wearing a tie, the tie came off. I drew a line in the sand and said, "no more." I received more than a handful of disapproving looks from the older attendees, but then, one day, I noticed that more residents, like me, were also going without a tie. Before long, it was the norm. I know I had a firsthand role in altering the hospital's consciousness regarding wearing a tie.

The truth is that the "rules" of this game called life are constantly evolving, not in a "right" versus "wrong" paradigm, but in conflicts of consciousness. With time, what once felt impossible or taboo can become normal, even celebrated. That's why living intentionally matters so much. Don't let yourself be an NPC in your own life, passively following society's script.

Instead, step back and reflect.

Consider the labels you accept and how you express love in your highest language. Ask yourself: "Which labels align with my true self, and which ones were handed to me?" Choose to break free from the unexamined codes that no longer serve you. Rewrite your story. Shape the energy you want to project into the world. Because ultimately, the life you live is your creation. If you still doubt this, look at your story, hold it up to a mirror, and take a few more **C.A.B. rides**.

RABBIT HOLE
GAIA Television – Regina Meredith, *Open Minds* and George Noory, *Beyond Belief*

CHAPTER 15

CRACKING OPEN YOUR SHELL

The knowledge I gained in medical school matters, and yet, it is incomplete.

Everything I learned was based on the physical, the macro, the observable. But since the 1920s, quantum physicists have studied a world smaller than electrons and protons, a tiny and counterintuitive realm that often seems like magic. This reminds us that when our energy and mindset shift, our biology changes too.

Let me take you back to the earliest chapter of my professional life. It's 2003, and I'm fresh out of residency, filled with ambition, and ready to make my mark. I had just signed on with a Family Medicine practice in South Lake Tahoe, California, and my wife and I were packing up to start our new adventure together. We found a cozy house at the foot of Echo Summit in a small area known to locals as Christmas Valley. It was straight out of a storybook. I was eager to plant roots in this picturesque town about to become our new home.

The practice I joined was unique, even by today's standards. Our group served about two-thirds of the town's 24,000 full-time residents, providing care for everything from births to hospice, and all the messy, beautiful moments in between. I wasn't just a family doctor; I delivered babies, assisted surgeries, and ran the hospital floor and the ICU. I even took extra shifts working the E.R. on the North Shore of Incline Village and worked as the local jail doctor. My colleagues liked to joke that they sent all their "asses" to me because I also handled colonoscopies and hemorrhoid care. I did it all, the full breadth of Family Medicine; that was me.

Our practice was bustling at its peak, with over 30 staff members and six doctors. My schedule was relentless. I saw around 30 patients daily, excluding my on-call time. As a young physician, I was determined to get everything just right. I followed protocols like clockwork, charted on time with detail, and ensured every task was perfect. "No one is going to die on my watch," I told myself. My goal was simple: be the ideal physician: always on time, prepared, and efficient. I took everything, every person, and every situation in my care as seriously as it should be, *to me*.

I prided myself on running a tight ship.

I listened attentively to my patients, communicated clearly with my nurses, and kept everything running smoothly. In hindsight, I had become somewhat of a robotic physician. This approach worked well; it kept my staff seemingly happy because they knew what to expect. It also prevented unnecessary chaos and made me feel like I was following every rule.

My wife stopped by the office one day before we headed out for lunch. While I was busy seeing patients, she wandered through the practice, introducing herself and chatting with my team. That evening, as we were lying in bed, she started laughing, a mischievous laugh I knew all too well. It was the kind of laugh that meant she was about to tease me, but in her usual loving way.

"So, I met your staff today," she grins. I braced myself, ready to hear about what a great doctor I was or how they admired my efficiency and professionalism. But instead, she hit me with something I didn't expect. "You know," she began, "they all think you're serious, tightly wound, and kind of distant."

That caught me off guard. "Really?" I asked, genuinely confused.

She nodded, her smile softening. "It's funny because you're one of the goofiest, most open people I know. But that side of you doesn't show at work. Maybe you should start sharing more of yourself with your staff, patients, and everyone."

Her words stuck with me. She was right. I had worked so hard to be the "perfect" doctor that I lost sight of my human side. I promised myself I'd never become one of those old-school, three-piece-suit doctors like my father's generation. I wanted to be open, vulnerable, and real, but my obsession with perfection had built walls around me. That night, I realized it was time to shift from just practicing the science of medicine to embracing the art of connection.

Like placing an order with the universe, the lesson I needed came to me the next day. A man in his early 30s walked into my office, visibly uncomfortable. He was struggling with obsessive-compulsive tendencies that were wreaking havoc on his marriage. His wife, also my patient, had practically dragged him in, and his body language said it all–he didn't want to be there. He sat across from me, arms crossed, all macho and stoic, his emotional walls as solid as granite. Just thinking about how I would soften the wall in front of me was intimidating.

If I wanted to help him, I'd have to find a way past his shell. But the truth was, I'd first need to crack open my own. Vulnerability isn't easy. It's messy, uncertain, and exposed, like cracking an egg. Once you break that shell, there's no going back.

I took a deep breath, and before I could second-guess myself, I did something I'd never done before. I cracked open my shell. "Look," I began, my throat suddenly dry. "I know what you're going through because I've been there too."

His expression didn't change, but I kept going. "I deal with OCD. I take Prozac. And, if I'm honest, it sometimes drives my wife up the wall."

The air suddenly felt heavy. His face turned pale, and my stomach clenched. Was I mistaken? Had I damaged my credibility as a doctor? The silence between us grew longer, and I mentally scolded myself for taking such a big risk.

Then, something remarkable happened. His eyes filled with tears. "I thought I was the only guy dealing with this," he said softly.

At that moment, the walls he'd built so carefully crumbled. He opened up about his struggles, his frustrations, and his fears. He thanked me profusely and promised to follow my advice. His vulnerability was the most unexpected gift, hitting me like a wave.

That connection transformed both of us. What could have taken months of clinical detachment to achieve happened in minutes. By cracking open my shell and taking the leap, I'd given him permission to crack open his shell and do the same. That's the Boomerang in action.

This patient became a long-term one, and later, his wife shared that their marriage had never been better. But that experience wasn't just a breakthrough for him, it was a revelation for me. I realized the transformative power of vulnerability in healing, not just for patients, but for myself as a physician and as a human being.

On the other hand, remaining stuck in negative patterns, as my patient had been, can create a significant ripple effect, not only on your well-being but also on the relationships and environments around you. His struggles were putting a strain on the most important relationship in his life: his marriage. It serves as a reminder of how one person's unresolved challenges can influence an entire dynamic, like the "bad apple effect," which demonstrates how a single negative influence can undermine the success and harmony of a team.

Let's discuss the "bad apple effect." This phenomenon demonstrates how much influence a single person can have on a team's success or failure. Research shows that teams with even one opposing member can see a 30-40% drop in productivity compared to teams without such a member. In fact, a team's overall performance is often best predicted by its least effective member. This means that one person's negativity not only affects them but can also spread throughout the entire group, significantly harming results and morale. In sports terms, this is akin to a coach commenting on whether a player helps create a positive locker room or not.

Better Health Starts with Better Thoughts

The experience of vulnerability taught me that I am not a physician first; I am a human being who *happens to be* a physician. Humans can't ignore the connection between thoughts and health and its impact on those around us.

Change starts with you.

From this day forward, I challenge you to be honest with yourself and others in every interaction. Hold up a mirror and look closely, not to judge but to observe with curiosity. Your perceptions, biases, and reality are all just beliefs, and beliefs influence health.

Until that day I cracked open my shell, I had been living in a story about what a doctor should be, a story shaped by my physician father's journey. My job was to follow in his footsteps and emulate his example. At the time, this seemed like the only roadmap to being a "good doctor."

But here's the truth: that story wasn't mine; it was his.

It was a patchwork of inherited beliefs and observations from my environment, stitched together by expectation rather than authenticity. Letting go of that story and releasing myself from the mold of the "ideal physician" were some of the most freeing moments of my life. That day, I became the doctor I had always aspired to be.

When I embraced my authenticity, everything changed. I stopped trying to fit into someone else's narrative and started showing up as myself. I let go of the inner conflicts that clashed with what my dad would see as ideal. That shift allowed me to connect more deeply with my patients, not just as their doctor but as a fellow human being. It made me more present with my family and even opened the door to meaningful conversations with strangers. Letting go of that story didn't just make me a better doctor; it made me a better version of myself.

RABBIT HOLE
Alpha Brainwave Training

CHAPTER 16

FROM KNOWLEDGE TO WISDOM

I'll never forget my first day of medical school. I returned to my dorm room that afternoon, utterly overwhelmed. In just one morning, we'd covered gross anatomy, biochemistry, histology, and physiology. Each lecture demanded mastery of four to six textbook chapters. My brain felt like an overstuffed filing cabinet about to burst, and the sinking realization hit me: "It's day one, and I'm already 16 chapters behind."

That moment nearly broke me.

I remember sitting on the edge of my bed, staring at my stack of books, wondering how I could keep up. My equally frazzled roommate looked at me and said what we were both thinking, "What did we get ourselves into?" We both stepped back and realized there were only two tests: the midterm and the final. We had all semester to absorb all this information, and instead of obsessing over keeping up, we could focus on genuinely learning one concept at a time.

That slight, intentional shift, from cramming to understanding, changed everything. I began to approach my studies differently, not as a race to memorize facts but as an opportunity to apply knowledge meaningfully and find the connections between each class I was taking. I started making audio cassette tapes that would bring the topics from each class into a unified picture. I would listen to them when I worked out, ate, and even fell asleep at night. I stopped chasing grades and realized this was about my future patients, not me. I began asking myself, "Why does this matter? How does it relate to the broader context? How will I apply this concept later?"

I didn't realize it at the time, but I was beginning to shift from being a consumer of knowledge to a creator of wisdom. It wasn't just about absorbing what was in the textbooks anymore; it was about synthesizing, questioning, and applying it to real-life scenarios. That approach not only made me a better student, but it also laid the foundation for the doctor I wanted to become.

Looking back, I chuckle at how daunting those "basic sciences" once seemed.

At the time, I believed the goal was to master every detail through rote memorization, but life has shown me that knowledge alone isn't enough. What really matters is how we turn that knowledge into wisdom. Wisdom is what we can use to truly connect, heal, question, and most importantly, grow.

As a physician, it means offering not just a diagnosis but a way forward. As a person, it means taking every lesson and challenge and finding a way to transform them into something meaningful. Dr. Joe Dispenza would put it a little differently, but eloquently, in a way that ties beautifully with Biological Decoding: "A memory without emotional attachment is called wisdom."

That first day of med school taught me one of the most important lessons: wisdom isn't about knowing everything, it's about understanding what matters and connecting the vital dots.

RABBIT HOLE
The Emerald Tablets

CHAPTER 17

WHAT WE RESIST PERSISTS

Jean, a 41-year-old woman, came to me to address her complex gut health, which had plagued her on and off for 20 years. Before seeing me, she had consulted countless GI specialists and alternative physicians. Over the years, she had undergone every conceivable diagnostic test, followed every type of diet, and experimented with various treatments, from traditional approaches to more obscure modalities.

When Jean walked into my office, she carried an air of determination, as if she were ready to rewrite her story. She'd adopted an immaculate diet: no wheat, gluten, dairy, or simple sugars. Yet, despite her discipline and sacrifices, her symptoms persisted. What struck me most that first day wasn't her list of dietary restrictions or her carefully researched supplements; it was how, in the very first conversation, she openly identified the real culprit behind her struggles. "It's stress," she admitted plainly, almost as if the words slipped out before she could stop them.

Still, Jean clung tightly to the idea of a physical solution. She was adamant about pursuing food sensitivity tests, stool studies, and more exhaustive workups all over again. "Let's rule everything out," she insisted, even though she had already taken that route. So, we did. As expected, the results revealed no significant findings.

Over the first year we worked together, her frustration grew. She'd find temporary relief from a new protocol or treatment, only for her symptoms to return, often worse than before. "I'm doing everything right," she would say, exasperated. **"Why is this still happening to me?"** Her restricted diet was exhausting her, and the endless search for answers was draining her spirit.

I knew that healing for Jean wasn't about another test or supplement. It was about helping her bridge the gap between what her body was telling her and what her heart and mind already knew. But as any doctor or person knows, people aren't ready to hear the truth until they are ready. My job wasn't to force it but to plant seeds gently.

During one of our quarterly appointments, I asked Jean a simple question that she seemed to dismiss each time I asked it before: "When are your GI issues the best for you?" For the first time, Jean hesitated. Then, almost reluctantly, she said, "Whenever I'm at our vacation home in Colorado, my symptoms disappear. Completely."

That was the crack in her shell I'd been waiting for.

Slowly, her resistance softened, and more pieces of her story began to emerge. She admitted she hated living in Austin and longed to move to Colorado, but her husband loved Austin, and their kids were deeply rooted in the community. Even more telling, she revealed that she could eat whatever she wanted during international travel, whether in South America, Africa, or Europe, without a single GI issue.

At that moment, I wanted to gently shake her and ask, "Why didn't you tell me this sooner?" But I understood why. She wasn't ready to connect those dots yet. So, I asked her a crucial question: **"If I could snap my fingers and fix everything instantly, what would it take to fully heal your symptoms?"** She answered immediately: "I would move out of Austin."

It was as if she'd been holding her breath for years and had finally exhaled. Her body wasn't just reacting to food; it was responding to a life she felt unable to digest. **Naming her truth, no matter how daunting, was transformative.** Though her external circumstances hadn't yet changed, her symptoms began to ease.

From then on, our work shifted.

Whenever her symptoms flared, I encouraged her to "visit" Colorado, either physically or mentally. I reminded her that the body doesn't distinguish between a real place and a vividly imagined one. Her body relaxed when she visualized herself surrounded by the peace and freedom she felt there, and her symptoms diminished. She reconciled that her conflict stemmed from her feelings about Austin and the fact that moving would be uprooting everyone else in her family who loved it.

Eventually, Jean took the hardest step: she had an honest talk with her husband. Together, they decided to revisit the idea of moving once their kids finished school. The compromise brought relief because a solution was in sight, and Jean had stayed true to her feelings and was heard.

Since then, I rarely hear from Jean. She no longer fixates on tests or treatments. Instead, she listens to her body, respects its signals, and aligns her actions with her inner compass.

Jean's story reminds me of a universal truth: the clearest way to describe 'stress' is a clash between our beliefs and someone else's, showing up as inner resistance and a disconnect between our body, mind, and intuitive spirit. The body always communicates with us, but modern medicine and society often teach us to block out its voice in favor of diagnostic labels and physical fixes. Still, when we feel "off," it's not a failure; it's a gift, an invitation to take a **C.A.B. ride.**

Healing isn't about fixing symptoms but listening to our stories first. And sometimes, all it takes to start that journey is the courage to stop resisting what persists and speak your truth.

RABBIT HOLE

Drake's Equation

CHAPTER 18

STILL NOT CONVINCED? LET'S LOOK AT DREAMS, HYPNOSIS, AND PSYCHEDELICS

Almost every year, like clockwork, I find myself trapped in a recurring dream–a nightmare. I've realized my dream is quite common, too. It's so widespread that it's called: **The Final Exam Dream**. Some of you might even recognize it immediately. The dream usually starts with me returning to high school or college, feeling those familiar first-day jitters. At first, everything seems normal, but then the bell rings, and I can't find my math class. Worse, I don't even have my schedule. The days begin to blur together, and I miss not just math, but *every* class. At first, I feel mild anxiety, nothing serious. But as the days go by, I start to panic. I ask people where my classes are, but no one knows. I don't see the teachers or the classroom numbers. The frustration builds until I finally find my math class on the day of the final exam. I sit down, the test paper is handed to me, and I realize I have no idea how to answer a single question. That's when I wake up, my heart pounding, overwhelmed with panic, feeling like a total dipshit.

But then, the fog of panic lifts as I realize it's just a dream, and relief washes over me. The tension in my body melts away, and I find myself reflecting on what just happened, because it's not just a random nightmare, it's something more meaningful: a symbolic message my mind is trying to communicate in dream form.

The part that truly strikes me about this dream isn't just the message it holds; it's how real it feels. The panic and anxiety are so vivid, as if my body can't tell the difference between the dream world and waking life. My thoughts trigger a biological response, my heart races, my breath shortens, and I feel overwhelmed. Even though I'm just lying there asleep, my body believes every part of it.

In psychology, Carl Jung, a renowned pioneer of dream analysis, believed that dreams are more than just strange, fleeting thoughts. He viewed them as a bridge between our conscious and subconscious minds. Jung stated, **"The dream is a doorway to the soul. Who looks outside, dreams; who looks inside, awakens."** In his perspective, dreams help us become whole. When they repeat, like my final exam dream, they often suggest something unresolved in our psyche that needs attention. I've also heard that this type of dream is more common among individuals with type A personalities, people who like to control their lives' outcomes. That makes no sense; I've never been told I am type A. (Ha!)

I've explored dream analysis myself, delving into the intriguing world where symbols, abstract events, and emotions intersect to create a map of our inner lives. It's almost as if the subconscious mind is trying to reach out through an umbilical cord, linking what we consciously experience with what's simmering just below the surface. However, unlike this dream example, most dreams appear nonsensical; and they are. They are filled with a wealth of symbolism. For example, Jung suggests that if you are a man, male characters may symbolize your inner self, while female dream characters represent external aspects. This is not universally agreed upon, but it is simply one example of how our mind communicates with us through symbols.

Biological Decoding is a conceptual framework that connects psychology with biology by integrating scientific research from fields like neurology, immunology, endocrinology, epigenetics, gene expression, and related disciplines. An experienced Biological Decoder recognizes that most thoughts operate subconsciously, making it challenging to trace a disease back to its emotional conflict without understanding how the mind conceals thoughts linked to deeply rooted emotions. **Often, it uses symbolism to hide these thoughts from our conscious mind, so we are not routinely aware of them.** However, when something triggers a current event, it can evoke strong emotions because the symbolism of the two events is often linked. These conflicts reside in the mysterious realm of subconscious thought, frequently symbolically, as in dreams, which adds to the complexity.

Since our mind generates symbols for thoughts, a subconscious thought tied to a powerful emotion can trigger the same biochemical response as a conscious thought. This means our biology can continue to manifest according to that symbol's meaning without knowing it if we have not done the inner work to release the emotional conflicts that trigger powerful negative emotions.

Take my ankylosing spondylitis, which mainly affects my lower spine, giving it a bamboo-like appearance on X-ray. Bamboo, known for its strength, has been used in home construction. While I wasn't consciously focused on carrying my father's conflicts my whole life, my subconscious mind stored emotional wounds as symbolic memories, just like it does with dreams. Since thoughts influence biology through symbols, my autoimmune disease reflects a deeper story and, because of its symbolic nature, was unconsciously triggered by conscious moments.

In Biological Decoding, my ankylosing spondylitis is connected to the conflict of "carrying a weight." My body biologically responded to support my mind's architectural symbolism by reinforcing my spine, both symbolically and physically, to carry a heavier burden. The good news is that if we can reshape our thoughts and perceptions of our story, we can change the negative energy we hold and restore our biology to health (or at least stop disease from advancing further).

This reflects the sentiment from the last chapter of my first book: **"Where thoughts go, Energy flows."**

We don't need to wait for the next recurring dream to show us what's out of alignment. We can look inward, reflect on the thoughts that drive profoundly negative emotions, and start to change the stories we tell ourselves. When we do, the energy we generate will shift, bringing us closer to healing, growth, and a life lived with intention. So, if there's one lesson from my recurring dream, it's this: Our thoughts are powerful. They shape how we feel whether they are real or imagined. Once we realize that, we can rewrite the script of how our thoughts influence the direction of our biology.

Hypnosis

Early in college, I attended an event that unknowingly sparked my fascination with the mind. My school had invited a hypnotist to entertain incoming first-year students. Although I had no intention of volunteering to go on stage, I was eager to watch the participants out of curiosity. He asked the volunteers, and anyone in the audience who wanted to participate from the comfort of their chair, to focus on his voice as he guided them into a state of relaxation. Looking back, I now understand that this was his way of inducing what's known as theta brain waves, a deep state of relaxation where the unconscious mind becomes more accessible.

By the end of the evening, I found myself at the center of attention in a way I hadn't expected. To my surprise, I became hypnotized and was brought onto the stage where I danced half naked and even spoke like a baby when he regressed me to a much younger age. The strange thing was that I had very little memory of what had happened, and I wasn't embarrassed when I was told what had taken place. I was amazed at how easily I slipped into hypnosis. I couldn't stop thinking about it. What was this mind-altering state? How did it work? Why was I so susceptible?

This experience occurred before the internet made everything easily accessible, so I turned to our campus library for answers. I devoured every book I could find on hypnosis, captivated by the idea that the mind could be unlocked this way. Eventually, I started practicing hypnosis with my friends. One session stood out to me- one that changed my entire view of the subconscious mind's power and ability.

Two of my friends, who had been in a relationship for five years, asked me to try age regression on them. I thought it would be fun, so I gave it a shot. Something extraordinary happened when I regressed my male friend back to the day he met his girlfriend. He wasn't just recalling that moment from memory; he was reliving it. He described the color of the shirt he was wearing, the floral details on her dress, the music artist whose song was playing in the background, and even the exact 10-minute joke he had told her that night. His girlfriend was amazed at how vividly he recalled everything, describing each detail in perfect clarity. It was truly remarkable; he was like a living tape recorder of a special moment.

The details were a little muddy when I woke him up and asked him to recall the joke. He could only remember bits and pieces, but the memory was crystal clear in that thoroughly relaxed, theta state. This moment revealed something profound to me: our brains hold onto every memory, every detail of our lives, even those we think we've forgotten. Those memories are stored in our subconscious, locked away and often seemingly unreachable, until something like hypnosis unlocks them.

What fascinated me even more was how deeply our memories are tied to emotions.

In that state, my friend wasn't just recalling facts about his first meeting with his girlfriend; he was reliving the excitement, the joy, and the nervousness of his first date with her. The emotions tied to that memory were as vivid and intense as they had been that day, years ago. It became clear that our memories don't just reside in the mind; they also reside in the subconscious of our body, waiting to be tapped. They stay with us, and the emotions attached to those memories can be triggered, sometimes unexpectedly, by outside events, sounds, smells, or even just a song tied to a memory.

How many of us have heard a song from our past and been

instantly transported to a specific moment? Suddenly, you feel the emotions of that moment flood back, whether it's joy, sadness, or something in between. It becomes so real you can practically taste it. Our minds and bodies are deeply connected in this way, holding onto the emotions of our past in ways we might not fully understand or assign meaning to.

But here's the thing: sometimes, an emotion surfaces–a sudden wave of fear, anger, or sadness–and we have no idea why it's there. It seems to come out of nowhere. This is precisely how PTSD works. An event, an experience, or even a specific sensation can trigger emotions that feel disconnected from the present moment, even though they're tied to a long-buried past trauma. It's not that the emotion is irrational; we just haven't consciously linked it to a belief filed in our subconscious.

This is where hypnosis can be transformative. Hypnosis provides a unique tool for bridging the gap between the subconscious mind and our conscious awareness. It allows us to access deeply-buried memories, fears, and emotions often hidden beneath the surface, untouched by our everyday awareness. By entering a relaxed state, we can gently bring these suppressed memories into the light and process them with greater clarity and control.

When we work with these memories in a safe, relaxed environment, we can transform them. Hypnosis offers a way to reframe and release the emotional charge associated with these memories, enabling us to form healthier, more positive associations with our past. It's not about erasing or forgetting the past; it's about shifting how we relate to it. By doing so, we can break free from subconscious (and sometimes irrational) fears and patterns that may hold us back in the present, paving the way for personal growth and emotional healing.

Ultimately, I learned from this experience that we are more than just our conscious thoughts. We are a complex web of memories, emotions, and experiences that live inside us—sometimes hidden, sometimes suppressed, but always there—ready to surface when we face them. Hypnosis is a valuable tool that can help us explore this inner world, unlocking the power of the subconscious mind to create lasting change. Whether through hypnosis, mindfulness, or meditation, the journey to healing involves acknowledging even the hidden parts of ourselves, embracing them, and allowing them to guide us toward greater understanding and lasting peace.

Meet Ray

Ray was a Marine: tough, resilient, and deeply proud of his service. He had been deployed five times, each tour testing the limits of his courage and pushing him further into the crucible of war. To everyone around him, Ray was a true warrior, the kind of guy who never flinched, never backed down, and someone you'd want in your corner in a dark alley. He was the embodiment of bravery and stoicism. But when he returned from his last deployment, something had changed. Beneath the hardened exterior, there was a quiet, crippling storm brewing inside him. It was palpable just being in his presence. He came to see me not as a broken man but as someone looking for answers–ones he was sure had to do with something physical. He had always been a man of action, never the type to succumb to weakness. But now, he found himself paralyzed by a dog barking. It wasn't just an annoyance or a momentary irritation; it was a trigger: a visceral, overwhelming flood of terror that overtook him in an instant. This simple sound brought him to his knees. Panic attacks, uncontrollable fear, and an intense desire to retreat from life were now his constant companions. It was complete incapacitation for him.

Ray was desperate for an explanation of a physical cause, something he could wrap his head around, something to be understood so that he could fight. He was convinced that something was wrong with his body. but I knew the truth ran more profound than that. This wasn't a physical ailment at all. It was the manifestation of the profound, unseen scars of war, the trauma that soldiers carry long after the battlefield fades from sight. But before I could ask him to consider the emotional and psychological roots of his condition, I needed to meet him where he was.

As I do with every patient, I began by addressing his physical symptoms, which he believed were the root cause. I talked to him about triggers, about how our bodies hold onto trauma, sometimes in the form of inexplicable panic. I gently planted seeds of understanding about the mind body connection and how, sometimes, the body can carry trauma even when the mind doesn't want to confront it.

It wasn't until I felt Ray was ready that I shifted the focus to the fundamental question: Why the sound of a dog barking? What was it about that specific sound that triggered such intense fear? Ray couldn't explain it. His mind was blocked, unwilling or unable to connect the dots at that moment. That's when I suggested he attend a retreat specifically designed for combat veterans with PTSD. This wasn't your average retreat; it involved the use of psychedelics, including psilocybin and 5MEO DMT, substances that had been gaining recognition for their potential therapeutic benefits in mental health, especially for people suffering from PTSD.

Now, I want to be precise. When I first heard about the use of psychedelics in mental health, I was the last person to even consider the idea. I had never touched any drug, not once. I was the kind of guy who would flush anything remotely recreational down the toilet, dismissing it as harmful or dangerous. But by the time I met Ray, I had come to understand something that had been outside my worldview for decades: certain psychedelics can pierce the psyche, allowing people to confront deeply-buried emotions and memories.

It wasn't until my late 40s that I began exploring the mental health benefits of psychedelics, challenging my own ingrained beliefs. I had grown up in the Nancy Regan era of "Just Say No," where any conversation about drugs was followed by shame and condemnation. But over time, I realized that psychedelics, like psilocybin, could serve as powerful tools for healing, especially for those struggling with PTSD. They can help individuals connect with the root causes of their trauma, allowing them to process and release the emotional weight that has been carried for far too long.

Ray wasn't hesitant to attend the retreat.

His pain was deep, and his suffering was reaching a breaking point. He was on the edge, battling suicidal thoughts, feeling like he couldn't escape the ghosts of his past. When he returned from the retreat, I saw a different Ray. There was a softness to him, a peace that hadn't been there before. He shared his experience with me, which was nothing short of profound.

Under the influence of psilocybin, Ray was shown the events of his last deployment, the one that had been the source of his trauma all along. He was leading a group of 10 men on a mission in the Middle East. As they approached their target, something felt off. Ray heard a dog barking. Trusting his instincts, he ordered his men to retreat, but it was too late. An IED exploded, killing his men. Ray was the only survivor. Until that day, Ray's conscious mind did not recall the preceding event of the dog barking.

The guilt that haunted him, the guilt of surviving when his brothers didn't, had been buried deep within him, unresolved and unacknowledged. It had manifested in response to a nearly inescapable sound, a dog barking, which triggered a flood of emotions tied to that moment: fear, loss, and an overwhelming sense of responsibility. But under the influence of psilocybin, Ray was finally able to see his origin story, the traumatic event that had been the root cause of his panic attacks.

Once he understood what had indeed happened and acknowledged the depth of his pain, he was able to release the guilt, the shame, and the anguish that had been driving his PTSD. The transformation was nothing short of remarkable. Since that moment, Ray has never experienced PTSD symptoms or panic attacks again, not even when he hears a dog barking.

The most potent part of Ray's story is that now, he's helping others.

He's become a warrior in a different way: a warrior for healing. He's passing his gift to other veterans, breaking the stigma around PTSD, and encouraging them to seek help. He's showing them a path to healing that doesn't rely on simply numbing the pain but rather understanding and confronting it directly. Ray is living proof that the fight doesn't end when you leave the battlefield; it's an ongoing journey. However, healing is possible with the right tools, support, and a willingness to face the past, often symbolically buried in our subconscious.

In the end, PTSD isn't just a set of symptoms; it's the body's way of holding onto trauma that has yet to be processed. It's not just about the mind; it's about the soul and the emotional scars that carry through time. With therapies like psychedelics, we're learning to confront our shadow selves to release the trauma and begin healing, not just veterans like Ray, but anyone who's experienced deep emotional wounds. It's about finding a way to stop running, avoiding, and finally face what's been buried so that we can truly heal.

RABBIT HOLE
Family Constellation Therapy

CHAPTER 19

How Our Brain's Organization Shows Us Where to Place a Temporary Roadblock

I've discussed the quantum energy behind our thoughts and emotions extensively, but now, let's focus on the hardware. Understanding the structure of our brain helps us understand why taking a **C.A.B. ride** with our thoughts can improve our health, relationships, and decision-making. While the brain is more complex than just three layers, simplifying it will make connecting with its workings easier.

Layer 1: The Reptilian Brain

Let's start with the brain's most primal function, the reptilian brain. Fortunately, we don't have to remind ourselves to breathe consciously, keep our heart beating, or manage blood sugar levels. These essential functions run automatically, even when unconscious, like in a coma.

Layer 2: The Limbic System

Next is the limbic system, our brain's emotional center, sometimes called the "mammalian brain." This system controls how we process emotions, adapt to experiences, pick up on social cues, and navigate motivation and rewards. It's closely tied to the lower brain's functions, like triggering the fight-or-flight response–the emotional and physical rush we feel when we face danger (or excitement).

The amygdala, your brain's emotional bodyguard, is at the core of the limbic system. It reacts quickly to scan for threats or rewards, triggering your fight-or-flight response when necessary. Think of it as the decision-maker that drives your reactions until the prefrontal cortex, the rational part of your brain, takes over around age 25 to help control those impulsive responses.

(You might not want to remember your impulsive decisions before age 25 but think about the last time you drank too much. Alcohol acts like a roadblock, shutting down the rational part of your brain.)

Layer 3: The Prefrontal Cortex

The third layer, the prefrontal cortex, is what makes you the CEO of you. It controls higher brain functions like critical thinking, long-term planning, and emotional regulation. This is where mindfulness and self-awareness live, enabling you to respond logically, especially in stressful situations.

The prefrontal cortex gives us space to pause and reflect rather than reacting impulsively, as the amygdala often urges. This ability to slow down and think through options separates us from survival-driven instincts. Fear-based reactions lose their hold when we act from this layer, and we can make better decisions. Unfortunately, many of my patients, especially those fearful of COVID-19, rarely relied on this part of the brain. Instead, they fell into emotional dysregulation, which triggered a mix of signals that weren't helpful for health and healing.

Taking a C.A.B. ride to identify the thought that sparked a strong emotion creates a temporary roadblock between the prefrontal cortex and the other two brain layers. This pause allows us to observe and choose our responses with awareness and intention.

Think of the typical advice not to shop when you're hungry. Hunger, a primal drive controlled by the reptilian brain, pushes us to eat for survival. However, it can also affect our rational decisions, leading us to make poor choices in the grocery store. That "hangry" feeling is a perfect example of how the reptilian brain can block the rational parts of our brain.

Similar roadblocks happen when we're sleep-deprived, in pain, using recreational drugs, or dealing with high insulin levels from poor eating habits. While I often address physical S.T.A.M.P. triggers in my patients first, primal instincts are designed to protect us and will override willpower.

The primary purpose of the C.A.B ride with our thoughts is to create a space between the prefrontal cortex and the other two layers <u>momentarily</u> so we can reason before we send out our boomerang.

RABBIT HOLE
Experiential Learning - Consider joining a plant-psychedelic retreat (within legal bounds and with trained counselors), or attending a meditation retreat with Dr. Joe Dispenza, or doing Alpha-Brain Wave training

CHAPTER 20

THE BODY SPEAKS

"The body keeps the score, if the memory of trauma is encoded in the viscera, in heartbreaking and gut-wrenching emotions, in autoimmune disorders and skeletal muscular problems, this demands a radical shift in our therapeutic assumptions."

—Bessel van der Kolk, *The Body Keeps the Score*

Meet Jake.

Jake was a 51-year-old male who prided himself on his physical health. He had been a patient of mine for many years. I had always known him to be incredibly disciplined, determined, and seemingly invincible, but then some time ago, everything changed.

Jake was diagnosed with a heart arrhythmia called atrial flutter, a condition where the upper chambers of the heart send out rapid electrical signals, causing it to pump excessively. He had never experienced anything like it before, and after undergoing several tests and an ablation procedure, he thought he was back on track. None of the tests gave him any clue as to why this was happening in the first place, but he was happy to feel normal again. His health seemed restored, and he even returned to enjoying one of his favorite pastimes, snow skiing.

However, our bodies communicate with us in other ways if we do not listen or address the most important question: What was the ongoing thought linked to an emotion that occurred within the 6 to 12 months before this event began?

A year later, Jake faced a new, unexpected challenge. He developed a strange, persistent itch all over his body, known as generalized pruritus, but when he first wrote to me, he called it a rash. No matter what he tried, nothing helped. He used everything from various creams and steroids to visits with dermatologists, and he even flew out to the Mayo Clinic. Determined to find an answer, he pursued every avenue, but still had no relief.

The itch disrupted his sleep, so Jake finally reached out to me. Since he had already seen multiple specialists, I decided to call him directly and hear his story so I could get a clearer picture.

After listening for about 15 minutes, I realized there was no actual visible rash, only overwhelming itchiness. Other than that, he felt fine. I asked why it took him so long to bring this up to me, and he admitted he did not think it was within my wheelhouse since it seemed like a skin issue.

This is a common misconception in medicine. With so many specialties, when a patient shows a symptom in a specific domain, whether the GI tract, skin, heart, kidneys, liver, or brain, they are quickly referred out to a specialist in that area. This ingrained bias creates a mindset where even physicians forget that the body is not a collection of separate systems, but a connected, holistic system made of energy.

I asked Jake the question I always ask my patients since learning Biological Decoding: What was happening in your life in the 6 to 12 months before this started? He hesitated. "Nothing," he replied almost too quickly. After more prompting, he finally admitted that just before all this began, he and his girlfriend had started in vitro fertilization to try to have a child.

As he spoke, everything in his tone revealed he was unhappy with it. I asked him directly, without sugarcoating, if he wanted a child. He answered, "I do not want to have a kid, and next week she is going to have fertilized eggs implanted in her." The words hit me like a ton of bricks. He had kept this truth to himself for months. Shocked, I asked, "Wait, you mean you started this process six months ago, and now she is getting implanted next week, and you do not want a child? Does she know this?"

His response carried shame. "We have a great relationship," he said. "She knows all my friends, and since she sold her house and moved in with me during COVID, I do not want to mess it up. She has built relationships with my friends' spouses, and I do not want to rock the boat."

Jake already had a son in his twenties from a previous relationship, while his girlfriend had none and sincerely wanted children. Six months before his atrial flutter incident in 2022, she had sold her belongings, moved from Texas to Colorado, and committed fully to him, a step they had not actually fully discussed. Once again, major decisions were made without him speaking up. Now, he was about to begin IVF, still holding back his true feelings. The timing was painfully obvious.

Jake had never shared this story with anyone until now.

His body was communicating in the only way it knew how. His symptoms, the itching, the disrupted sleep, the physical response to emotional stress, reflected his inner struggle. His subconscious had carried the weight of this secret, and his body had found a symbolic way to express it. Out of fear of upsetting his girlfriend and avoiding conflict about children or moving in together, his body created a new biological response that mirrored his inner turmoil.

1. **Atrial flutter** symbolizes the emotional conflict of "I cannot let people in through the front door, and I do not have the freedom of movement." This matched when his girlfriend moved in without discussion during the

pandemic.

2. **Generalized pruritus** symbolizes something eating us up inside. The thought of having another child he did not want was consuming him.

I made it clear to Jake that he could not allow the IVF procedure to move forward without first facing his feelings. His girlfriend deserved honesty, and Jake needed to acknowledge his truth. He agreed. The next day, he finally sat down with her and voiced what he had hidden for more than six months.

A week later, I checked in. Jake told me the conversation went better than expected, and he felt enormous relief. Almost as an afterthought, he said, "Oh, and my itch resolved almost immediately. I have slept great every night since then." It was as if several bricks had been lifted from his back. His physical symptoms, which had tormented him for months, disappeared overnight.

What struck me was how unimpressed Jake seemed by this dramatic change despite seeing so many specialists. He had been so focused on physical causes that he had not stopped to notice the emotional trigger. His itch had been a biological symbolic symptom, a cry for help, and once the emotional burden was lifted, his body returned to balance.

Jake had been stuck in his limbic and reptilian brain for so long that he had built a roadblock, preventing him from using his cortical brain to connect the dots between conflict and biology.

While Jake experienced what looked like a miraculous recovery, I worried he might miss the deeper lesson his body was trying to teach. His dismissal of the emotional connection raised concern that the next time he withholds his truth, his body will again create distracting symptoms. I expect a call from Jake in the future, but I will be more prepared to help him face his inner truths.

Jake's story highlights intuitive truths I have seen many times in Biological Decoding. Once he acknowledged his conflict, he could not unsee it. That is the first step toward healing. He also took the second step, confronting his fear, sitting with his uncomfortable truth, and sharing it with the person he conflicted with.

Still, I worry he may miss the final key. If he does not fully release his conflict, his body will continue to speak, trying again and again to resolve what remains unresolved. His struggle will be in voicing his truths in the future, and if he fails, his body will once again create symbolic biology to "speak" what his mind is too afraid to confront.

Despite the time, money, and effort spent on doctors, Jake still feels more comfortable dismissing the importance of emotions. He may continue to experience dysfunction as long as he suppresses his truths, and his body will remind him of this until he learns that balance cannot be found any other way.

This time, I celebrated the win on my own..

RABBIT HOLE
Medical Intuitive

CHAPTER 21

THE BUSINESS OF HEALTH VS. THE BASICS

A closer look at advances, efforts, and expenditures in the American healthcare model reveals that much of it focuses on the final weeks of life. It has become a system more about battling time than about living well throughout the years we have.

I spent many years as a hospitalist, and during that time I saw firsthand the aggressive measures used to prolong life in its final moments. These included TPN (nutrition delivered through an IV), intubation to assist with breathing, and even surgical procedures aimed at extending life, sometimes only by a few days or weeks. It was heartbreaking to watch patients, often unknowingly, choose these drastic steps thinking they could buy just a little more time, only to pass away in a hospital room or aftercare facility instead of in the comfort of their own home, surrounded by loved ones.

While I understand the reasons for choosing these interventions, my years as a Medical Hospice Director gave me an invaluable perspective on the true nature of life's end, a perspective worth repeating. I observed two distinct types of people: those who were at peace with their lives, content with the love, joy, and experiences they had accumulated, and those who fought desperately for every breath, clinging to life despite their suffering, consumed by fear, regret, or unresolved conflicts.

No one in their final days wished they had worked more. Instead, they wished they had loved more deeply, lived more fully, and made peace with the natural flow of life, which only comes through the weeding of our emotional landscape.

This truth leads to a key point: health, especially emotional health, is the foundation on which everything else depends. More than anything, the mind influences our biology, relationships, and even financial well-being. To build a successful life, we must understand the connection between our conflicts and our bodies.

Recently, I saw some friends wearing patches they claimed could convert light energy into wave energy, helping stem cell regeneration. I am fascinated by technologies that operate at the deepest energy levels, from quantum particles to the influence of thought on cells.

My friends asked if I wear these patches, and while I was intrigued by the concept, I explained that I do not sell them. I sensed they wanted me to vouch for them, but as I often tell my patients, I always prioritize the fundamentals—those timeless practices that science repeatedly proves are the foundation of well-being. Once the fundamentals are established, and if someone still needs an extra nudge in a certain area, I am more than happy to explore other tools, including technological devices. Too often, however, I see the opposite happening: healthcare providers or industry figures pushing technology over the basics.

Here is my why.

If we could bottle the essentials, exercise, purpose, sex, and meaningful relationships, and put them in a single pill, it would cut down illness and death by at least 95 percent. This isn't just an empty claim but one backed by research, including the Blue Zones I mentioned earlier, where people consistently live to be over 100 years old.

When we live with purpose, joy, and community, we unlock our human superpowers that transform. That power comes from shifting harmful emotions and beliefs into love, peace, and gratitude. It is a change in perspective, a rewiring of our mental and emotional states that deeply impacts our biology and our lives.

When we connect to the overlying quantum field, the fabric of all, based on Quantum Field Theory, we are, in a sense, plugging into the Source of energy that imparts our superhuman capacity to self-heal and expand our perceived limited senses.

Just as a belief charged with strong emotion can powerfully alter our biology, that same force can limit us when we lack belief in ourselves and our innate, even superhuman, capacities. As Gregg Braden beautifully explains, we often depend on external technology while neglecting the "soft technology" built within us. Neuroscience calls it neuroplasticity—the brain's ability to rewire. I see it as our natural capacity for grey thinking: the art of holding multiple truths at once.

National Geographic explorer and author Dan Buettner produced an excellent documentary, Live to 100: Secrets of the Blue Zones, released in 2023. It is available on Netflix, and I highly recommend it if you are new to the concept.

In these Blue Zones, such as Okinawa in Japan, Sardinia in Italy, and Nicoya in Costa Rica, we find some of the longest-living populations on Earth. They do not live longer because of access to advanced medicine or new technology. They live longer because they value health, community, purpose, and love. Their days are active, their ties are strong, and their lives carry purpose beyond personal achievement. They tend gardens, care for family, and support each other through every stage of life.

It is not about external solutions, miracle pills, or light patches. It is about internal transformation. Health is an ongoing, creative process in these communities. People do not wait for health to fail before they act; they make daily choices that enhance their well-being and nourish body, mind, and spirit. In doing so, they create lives rich in meaning and purpose that last long after careers and social labels fade.

Longevity medicine and its research are advancing our understanding of health and medicine significantly, but I advise people to ask themselves what energy drives their thoughts. Is their belief in longevity meant to serve their "one thing" longer or is it rooted in a fear of dying?

We each hold the power to create that same life with a body built for longevity.

Our mindset is the foundation of health and happiness. When we cultivate a mindset rooted in love and purpose, we tap into an extraordinary energy that shapes every aspect of life. Instead of talking only about the mind-body connection, we must expand the discussion to the mind-organ connection, real and powerful, influencing not only physical health but also emotional well-being, relationships, and even financial prosperity.

I cannot stress enough that the key difference between most mind-body discussions and Biological Decoding is that Biological Decoding provides a thought framework that demonstrates how emotional conflicts influence our biology within specific organs through symbolic gene expression hidden within our subconscious. Therefore, tapping it takes deep inner work that moves beyond our mere conscious mind.

The key to health and happiness is not found in the latest gadgets or the most expensive treatments. It is not something to chase. It is within us, revealed by resolving our deepest emotional conflicts and holding onto the transformative energy of love, gratitude, and peace. This is the foundation of a true "health is wealth" mindset– the recognition that a long, fulfilling life always stems from thoughts connected to deeply rooted emotions, also known as our beliefs.

RABBIT HOLE
Connie Kaplan The Invisible Garment

CHAPTER 22

WHAT IS THE SUBCONSCIOUS?

Aristotle once said, **"Knowing yourself is the beginning of all wisdom."** A simple statement, yet profound. All wisdom begins within, and understanding ourselves is the key to unlocking growth and deepening our connection with others. Perhaps Aristotle already knew that true self-knowledge reaches far beyond the conscious mind.

Think of the subconscious mind like your smartphone. When you buy a new iPhone, it is blank, waiting for apps and settings. The more apps you download, the more it can do, but the more memory it consumes. Your mind works the same way. At first, when you learn something new like driving, you are hyper aware of every detail. That is your conscious mind. But with practice, the subconscious quietly takes over. You no longer think about every step, the program just runs in the background.

My wife and daughter love to tease me about this. I will often drive home lost in thought, completely oblivious to what is happening around me. One afternoon, my wife spotted a Great Dane wandering in the middle of our street. Fearing it might get hit, she pulled over, hazards flashing, and somehow managed to wrangle this horse-sized dog into her little four-door sedan. Moments later, they pulled into the driveway right behind me. Out jumps this giant dog while they laugh hysterically.

"You had to have driven right by us," my wife said. "You didn't notice the massive dog we were stuffing into the car 20 seconds ago?"

Nope, not a clue. Picture it: hazards blinking, traffic blocked on my actual street, my wife and daughter wrestling a Great Dane into a compact car, while I cruise past like a self-driving Waymo. To this day, they make it a game to see if I notice them on the road. I am proud to report I now see them about 40 percent of the time. Progress.

That story perfectly illustrates consciousness versus subconsciousness. My conscious brain was floating off in daily thought, while my subconscious ran the driving program. It kept me safe between the lines, but it sure was not paying attention to details.

It is a lot like *The Matrix*, when Neo downloads combat techniques. At first, it requires focus, but eventually the subconscious automates the moves. This is how we learn everything we repeat: driving, working, speaking, cooking. Once embedded, these programs hum along smoothly in the background.

As I mentioned earlier, Dr. Bruce Lipton, a former professor and research scientist, expanded our understanding of this in his book, *The Biology of Belief*. In the 1970s, his research challenged the long-held belief that genes and DNA rigidly determine our biology. Instead, he showed that DNA is influenced by signals outside the cell, what we now call epigenetics. These signals include everything from nutrients to stress to the energetic impact of thoughts and emotions.

Lipton's work revealed something powerful.

Our biology is not fixed. We can reshape it by changing how we think and what we believe.

He also highlighted the enormous capacity of the subconscious, noting that it has up to a million times more processing power than the conscious mind.

Sit with that for a moment.

The average person has 40,000 to 60,000 thoughts each day, most of which are guided by the subconscious. Even something as simple as thinking, *"I need to go to the bathroom,"* depends on subconscious programming learned long ago. As a toddler, you had to learn not to go in your pants, then master standing up, and eventually walking to the toilet–each step a separate program linked together. As an adult, it feels like one thought, but it's dozens of automated steps from several individual thoughts.

Here is the catch. The subconscious does not just store skills. It also stores our emotional conflicts, which form our beliefs. When your beliefs clash with someone else's, alarm bells go off. That is when the ego steps in.

The ego's job is simple: to protect you from pain.

Emotions act like a stoplight. Most of the time, we cruise on green. A hint that something feels off turns the light yellow. But when you get triggered, it is like your car slamming on the automatic brakes at a red light, your whole system jolts with whiplash. Learning to notice those red lights buried in your subconscious is the first step to healing.

When I turned 50, I gave myself a gift: a two-year Life Sabbatical. I revisited every major choice I had ever made to ask, "Were these truly my decisions, echoes of other people's expectations, or simply early programming?" What I thought would be reflective turned out to be profoundly disruptive, humbling, and at times almost unbearable. Yet it was essential. I was diving deep into my subconscious, rewiring beliefs that no longer served me.

I learned that when we clash with others, **it is often not "us** against them," but "ego against ego." Both are trying to protect, no matter the cost. The more we dismantle old, unhelpful beliefs, the less the ego rules us. And when the ego is gone, conflict no longer takes root inside us. That, I realized, is the beginning of inner peace.

The big question is, how do you heal something that feels out of reach from your conscious mind? During my sabbatical, I worked with four different therapists at once, seeking different perspectives for myself and for my patients so I could later explain it to others. I returned to something I had learned during my hypnosis training: the body and mind never forget; everything is stored within us, we just need the right tools to access it.

So, I tried everything I could. Hypnosis, psychedelic plant retreat, alpha brainwave training in Sedona, past life regression, EMDR, brain spotting, CBT, IV ketamine therapy, Enneagram work, sound therapy, and a seven-day meditation retreat with Dr. Joe Dispenza, to name a few. Each modality gave me a different doorway into my subconscious. **I started by focusing on my red lights.** For me, many of them were connected to my dad. Not because my dad was bad or wrong, but because the beliefs I had downloaded from him as a child no longer aligned with the adult beliefs I had developed. The clash created emotional red lights, and my ego responded with whiplash.

This leads to a critical understanding.

We experience three predominant states of consciousness in life, each often associated with distinct brain wave patterns. From birth until about age seven, our brains primarily operate in **Delta** waves (0.5 to 4 Hz) and **Theta** waves (4 to 8 Hz), slow, absorptive states linked with deep sleep and imagination. Children in this window are sponges, soaking up everything without filters. **Words, actions, and emotional tones are downloaded <u>directly </u>into the subconscious, shaping lifelong beliefs.**

Around age seven, the brain shifts toward **Alpha** waves (8 to 12 Hz), a calm but alert state that blends imagination with conscious thought. By adolescence, **Beta** waves (12 to 30 Hz) dominate, promoting logic, problem solving, and focus, but also increasing stress and racing thoughts.

In adulthood, we mostly stay in Beta, with Alpha, Theta, and Delta reserved for relaxation, creativity, meditation, or sleep. People in their 20s and 30s often live almost entirely in Beta, focused on building careers, relationships, and financial stability. It's like me driving past my family wrangling a horse-sized dog into a car, fully automated but not really present. Add social media distractions, and it's no wonder people of all ages get stuck in Beta.

By our 40s and 50s, we usually feel more comfortable in our external world, but that comfort often comes with a price. We begin to slow down, rediscovering reflection, creativity, and presence. This phase often coincides with midlife crises, which are really conflicts between old subconscious programmed beliefs and the adult beliefs we have formed. People often say they feel too old for an identity crisis, but I remind them that they are right on schedule. Every time the subconscious hits the brakes at a red light, it means you are ready to face it.

This progression can be viewed as a dance through brainwave states, moving from unfiltered absorption to effort and analysis, then to reflection, and finally, wisdom. The goal is to observe every emotional red and yellow light with curiosity, not judgment. Walk through the emotion, rather than around it. Once you notice the weed in your subconscious garden, you can't unsee it. Pulling that weed (rewiring your brain) is the empowering part, and using tools like meditation, therapy, or breathwork becomes a playground for growth.

Over time, I began to see the subconscious as a garden. At first, every weed you pull seems to bring up two more. But with consistent effort, it shifts from overhaul to maintenance. Like any garden, you plant seeds, pull weeds, water, and provide light. For the psyche, **meditation is the steady nourishment** that helps all other forms of healing take root.

Growing up Catholic, meditation carried a shadow for me. I had absorbed my father's belief that prayer was the only acceptable path to God, and meditation was "the work of the devil." I never questioned that belief until much later, and when I first tried meditation, I felt hesitation. That hesitation was not spiritual, it was programming. My subconscious attached meditation to betrayal of Catholicism and my father.

When I learned that meditation shifts brain waves into Alpha (8 to 12 Hz), Theta (4 to 8 Hz), and even Gamma (30 to 100 Hz), where the quantum field of possibility resides, I began to rewire my programmed belief about meditation. What once triggered shame and guilt became linked to wonder, peace, and love.

At first, I often told myself that my ADD brain couldn't meditate or that I was doing it wrong. Then I came across Jay Shetty's book, *Think Like a Monk*. He wrote, "Meditation is not broken when you are distracted; it is broken when you let yourself pursue the distracting thought." That changed everything. Meditation isn't about perfection but about gently bringing attention back, like a gardener tending to a stubborn patch of earth.

Around that time, I also discovered **Emily Fletcher's work**, a former Broadway actress who once struggled with crippling insomnia that made her physically ill. Meditation changed her life so profoundly that she left Broadway, sold everything, moved to India, and trained for three years before founding **Ziva**

Meditation. Her story captivated me. When I later took her course, I understood why. She explained meditation not as mysticism but as mechanics, making it accessible and life-changing. Today, about 90 percent of my patients have at least tried to meditate, and they notice the difference immediately if they skip a session, just like the body feels off when you miss a workout or a meal.

After two years of steady meditation and therapy, I had cleared many of the most enormous emotional weeds from my subconscious garden. Each practice I tried, from hypnosis to brain spotting to sound therapy, gave me a tool for clearing ground and planting something new. I am not finished, but my goal is removing every one of them.

Every weed I remove allows more light, clarity, and balance. The process has also deepened my compassion for my patients because I see in their struggles the same tangled weeds that I have had to pull out myself. At its core, we all long for the same thing: a peaceful garden.

When it is all said and done, our beliefs are not about seeking agreement with others or trying to change the minds of those who believe differently. The goal is to look in the mirror and clear our own emotional landscape. When we finish this work, we have essentially removed the garden's overseer, the ego.

No ego means no internal conflicts.

No internal conflicts means no emotional dysregulation.

No emotional dysregulation means we respond to others with love in our hearts, no matter what they believe.

That is peace on earth, and biology in perfect alignment with the mind.

RABBIT HOLE
Dr. Teresa Bullard, The Modern Mystery School

CHAPTER 23

THE COSMOS WITHIN: A JOURNEY INTO THE UNIVERSE THAT IS YOU

Imagine looking up at the night sky, marveling at the galaxies and stars scattered across the cosmic expanse, each a radiant masterpiece of energy and matter. Now imagine flipping that vision inward, peering into the intricate universe within your body. An undeniable reflection emerges: the grand forces shaping galaxies mirror the complicated systems that sustain life within you. The macrocosm of the Universe and the microcosm of the human body are not separate but deeply interwoven, operating under the same universal principles.

Hermes Trismegistus, the ancient sage of wisdom, revealed a timeless truth in the Hermetic Principle, **"As above, so below, as below, so above."** This phrase indicates an interconnectedness between the grand infinite workings of the cosmos and the detailed, intricate nature of the human experience. The principle refers to the idea that the patterns, energies, and laws that govern the vast Universe above also influence the microcosm within us below.

The Universe, as vast and awe-inspiring as it is, represents an intricate tapestry of space, time, energy, and matter. It encompasses everything from swirling galaxies to glowing stars, orbiting planets, and celestial bodies on a nearly incomprehensible scale. Yet when we reverse the lens of exploration and peer inward, we discover something equally profound, a universe within ourselves. Just as the cosmos stretches across infinite expanses, the human body unfolds its own intricate microscopic symphony of life, reflecting the same fundamental principles.

A galaxy of cells exists on a grand scale, with galaxies made up of billions of stars, gases, and dust that act as self-contained systems, orbiting their centers and adding to the larger structure of the Universe. On a microscopic level, our bodies contain trillions of cells, each functioning as a complex and intricate system. A single cell, much like a galaxy, has diverse parts: the nucleus as its core, organelles as its stars, and mitochondria as its powerhouses, all working together to maintain balance and support life.

The cell's membrane functions like dark matter for a galaxy; it maintains structure while enabling interaction with the environment. Just as galaxies vary in shape, size, and function, so do cells–each uniquely adapted for their roles within the larger organism. This symmetry between the macrocosm and microcosm is no coincidence; it reflects the fundamental unity of all existence.

Shared Elements: Cosmic vs Cellular Life

The connection between the Universe's macrocosm and the body's microcosm goes beyond their structural similarities. Both are built on a common foundation of elemental life. The same core elements, carbon, hydrogen, oxygen, and nitrogen, energize the stars and make up 99 percent of the human body. From the vastness of space to the tiniest cells, these elements are the fundamental building blocks of existence.

Yet, the parallels go deeper still.

At the atomic level, the Universe and our bodies are governed by the same quantum elements. The smallest particles—quarks, gluons, and leptons—are the building blocks of all matter. Their precise, repeating fractal patterns control the interactions of energy and mass, bridging the gap between science and the ancient wisdom that proclaims, "As above, so below, as below, so above."

The New Frontier of Healing, Honoring the Universe Within

We stand at a crucial moment where ancient wisdom meets advanced science, offering a revolutionary approach to health and healing. By seeing ourselves as energetic beings connected to the cosmos, we move beyond merely treating symptoms to restoring inner harmony, healing shifts from external treatments to aligning with the energy flow that sustains life. This starts with looking at our beliefs so we can achieve emotional regulation and inner peace.

Remember this: you are not just a collection of organs and systems; you are a universe in motion, governed by the same forces that shape galaxies and stars. Treat your body with the reverence it deserves, and you will discover a profound transformation. You unlock the infinite potential to heal, grow, and thrive by nurturing the energy within and appreciating the framework of thought called Biological Decoding, which makes it easier to see how disease at the organ level stems from deeply embedded emotional beliefs.

RABBIT HOLE
Reiki Energy Healing

CHAPTER 24

THE MEDICAL INTUITIVE:
A NEW LENS ON HEALING, A CASE FOR WHY
AI WILL NOT REPLACE PHYSICIANS

In 1965, researchers discovered the cosmic microwave background radiation, an invisible remnant of the Big Bang. Before this breakthrough, the idea of a universe born from a singular explosion was dismissed by many as speculation. Yet this unseen force, detectable only through specialized instruments, became evidence that forever reshaped our understanding of the cosmos.

"The most beautiful thing we can experience is the mysterious. It is the source of all true art and science."
—**Albert Einstein**

Just as uncovering our origin story transformed cosmology, a deeper understanding of the unseen aspects of ourselves can transform how we practice medicine and approach healing. It also opens the door to insights that connect directly to the idea of *The Disease of Belief.*

With that in mind, let's talk about the medical intuitive.

A medical intuitive is someone who claims to perceive information about a person's physical, emotional, or spiritual health through intuitive, non-traditional means rather than conventional medical testing. At first glance, this may sound outrageous, I understand, but hopefully it seems less so now.

In fact, research suggests there is more to this than meets the eye. As humans, we have the capacity to sense emotional energy in ways AI cannot. This reinforces the idea that disease is stored in the body as energy, something that can only be intuitively perceived.

A 2020 study published in the *Journal of Integrative and Complementary Medicine* titled "**Accessing the Accuracy of Medical Intuitives: A Subjective and Exploratory Study,**" reported remarkable accuracy among medical intuitives. This exploratory study examined trained intuitives who used visualization and intuition to scan the body and energy systems. Sixty-seven adults participated in standardized phone or video sessions in which medical intuitives shared their perceptions without dialogue. Participants later submitted anonymous evaluations. Results revealed striking levels of perceived accuracy: 94% for identifying a primary health issue, 100% for secondary issues (among respondents), 98% for describing life events, and 93% for linking life events to health concerns.

Just as cosmic background radiation is invisible yet carries profound truths about the universe, the insights from medical intuition remind us that not all truths can be detected by our five senses. Some are felt, sensed, or known, and when honored, they reshape our understanding of health and healing. Never underestimate your innate gifts, which cannot be measured by science alone. And never underestimate those who can sense the disharmony of your emotions as they impact your biology.

This study highlights that health extends beyond physical symptoms. It involves a dynamic interplay of past experiences, emotional states, and energetic imbalances. To uncover the root causes of illness, we must look beyond what is happening in the body today and examine unresolved issues from the past. Traumas, whether big or small, rarely vanish. They leave their imprint and often resurface later as physical illness.

When mind and body fall out of harmony, internal conflict arises. This imbalance eventually manifests physically. Our biology responds to our thoughts and emotions, making it essential to maintain a positive mental and emotional outlook. When negative feelings surface, the healthiest response is not suppression but acknowledgment, processing, and resolution. As you've learned, this means taking a C.A.B. ride with your thoughts, checking in regularly to prevent repression from becoming illness.

Meditation and other reflective practices are invaluable here. They create space to witness and integrate emotions, restoring balance and alignment. Healing often requires stepping back and consciously reverse engineering: ***What are the thoughts behind my emotions?***

Our bodies are both fragile and remarkably resilient.

True healing emerges when we recognize the dynamic relationship between mind, body, and energy, and how unresolved emotional wounds reverberate through our biology. Healing is less about silencing symptoms and more about listening to the story they tell. Thoughts are not fleeting whispers; they are architects of biology, shaping immune responses, gene expression, and even the energy fields surrounding us.

Just as Galileo dared to challenge the paradigm of his day and transformed humanity's view of the cosmos, we too are called to look beyond reductionist medicine. Illness is not solely chemical or genetic; it is experiential, emotional, and intensely energetic.

When we honor this truth, we see every thought as a seed. Some grow weeds, other wildflowers, but all shape the landscape of our health. By tending our inner garden with meditation, awareness, and courage to face what lies beneath, we cultivate not only longevity but also peace through emotional regulation.

The body never forgets, but it does forgive when given the right conditions to heal. The most powerful condition we can create is harmony between belief and spirit. When aligned, healing is no longer a mystery; it becomes the natural state of being.

RABBIT HOLE

Gregg Braden – Bridging Science, Spirituality, and the Real World

CHAPTER 25

THE ENERGY PARTY

Let's wrap up this book not with a lecture, but with a celebration. I call it an **Energy Party**.

Here's how it works: review your entire list of phone contacts. Go through each name and notice how each person makes you feel. Do not overthink it. Feel their name. If a name sparks the strongest feelings of love, gratitude, or peace, add it to your party list.

But here's the rule: this list isn't about who you typically invite out of habit, family duty, or social obligation. It's not about age, gender, status, or who's fun at a Friday night barbecue. This list is solely based on energy, considering how it influences your inner state. When you remove the usual filters and focus purely on resonance, you'll be surprised who makes the cut and who doesn't.

Once you've made the list, invite these people to the most unique gathering they've ever attended. Tell them why they were chosen. Trust me, people light up when they hear why they inspire love, gratitude, or peace in you.

Now for the next step.

Set the space. Create an environment that feels intimate, safe, and enjoyable, where distractions are minimal and where connection can be the primary focus. Let your guests know that there will be no small talk, no "what do you do for a living?" Instead, when introducing themselves, each person begins with:

1. What energy story brought them and the host, that is you, together? What experience sparked the connection between you?

2. What makes their soul come alive?

This instantly shifts the tone. You move out of superficial chatter and into conversations that open hearts through lived experience. From there, invite them to share the moments or practices that bring them into their highest energy.

The purpose is for each guest to connect with one person they don't know, ask these two questions, and then go back to the group to share what they learned about each other. Yes, you share the other person's story with the group. In doing so, the whole circle is brought together through an exchange of stories rooted in love, gratitude, and peace, and it keeps you engaged in actively listening at the same time. The outcome is a mutual gathering unlike anything you've ever experienced. Since these are all people you vibe with at the highest level, the others will likely vibe with them too.

There is genuinely no party like an **Energy Party.**

I've done this twice, and people still talk about them. Why? Because the more we connect with our highest self, both internally and with others, the more we progress in what I call the Ph.D. program of Wellness. This is the deeper curriculum of life through authentic connection. And here is where I leave you, full circle, at the doorway to the core message of this book. The greatest enemy of human potential is not genetics, not circumstance, not even environment. It is the unconscious prison of our own assumptions, what I have called throughout this work: **The Disease of Belief.**

Belief, when left unexamined, traps us in superficial conversations with life. It confines us to roles, labels, fears, and borrowed stories. But belief, when questioned, expanded, and transformed, becomes energy–energy that heals, changes, creates, and ultimately transforms us.

May your future gatherings, whether with a group or in your own inner dialogue, be Energy Parties of the highest kind. May you choose resonance over routine, connection over convention, love over fear, and may your inner force always reflect your most authentic self. Recognize that no one owes you anything. You earn the boomerangs in your life.

I'll leave you with two fascinating rabbit holes to explore, where you start embracing living with quantum thinking. Instead of responding like a passive NPC by calling something "crazy," adopt the mindset: "I don't know, but I am open to learning more." Be comfortable challenging your own beliefs. Be comfortable with being wrong.

RABBIT HOLE
Dark Matter and "Junk" DNA

About the Author

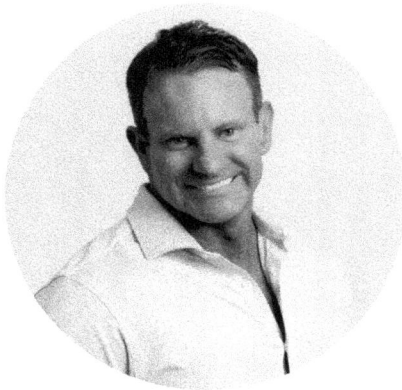

Kevin Hoffarth, MD, IFMCP is a physician, author of Functional Medicine: The New Standard, and the founder of BioFIT Medicine in Austin, TX, a concierge practice dedicated to transforming the way we understand health, illness, and the self. He integrates Functional Medicine, somatic awareness, identity psychology, and consciousness science to help patients reconnect with their inner coherence. He has a wife, daughter, two furry pets, and ten adopted fish. Learn more about his work at biofitmedicine.com.